Designing Robots to Improve Quality of Life for Older Adults

With adults over 60 becoming an ever-increasing proportion of the global population, the challenge of accommodating the needs, preferences, and abilities of this heterogeneous population has increased. One such method is with robots, which can be used to support everyday activities for older adults and enhance their quality of life. Older adults have been found to be quite open to the idea of interacting with robots, albeit with preferences for the nature of the task they want the robots to do. This book provides a comprehensive state-of-the-art review of the topic of designing robots for older adults.

This book translates research on aging, human factors, and human–robot interaction (HRI) into guidance that will be usable for practitioners who design robots for a range of applications. It offers a framework for HRI with a focus on personal characteristics, robot functionality, task demands, and interaction context. The application of this HRI framework for older adults provides the basis for this book. It covers the fundamentals of aging, a review of the different types of robots available now and in the future, the known facilitators and barriers for adoption, and the potential of robots for different everyday activities including social engagement, health and wellness, home maintenance, and security. Throughout, the authors emphasize the need to follow fundamental human factors processes and participatory design approaches that engage older adults in the design process, thus rendering the reader a thorough and contemporary understanding of robots as an essential future for assisting an aging population.

Designing Robots to Improve Quality of Life for Older Adults is intended for a broad professional audience, especially the design community, gerontologists, and human factors/ergonomics practitioners. It will also be suitable for students at the undergraduate and graduate levels as a supplementary textbook for courses in human factors, design for aging, and HRI.

Human Factors and Aging Series

Series Editor:
Wendy A. Rogers
University of Illinois Urbana-Champaign

Given the worldwide aging of the population, there is a tremendous increase in system, environment, and product designs targeted to the older population. The purpose of this series is to provide focused volumes on different topics of human factors/ergonomics as they affect design for older adults. The books are translational in nature, meaning that they are accessible to a broad audience of readers. The target audience includes human factors/ergonomics specialists, gerontologists, psychologists, health-related practitioners, and industrial designers. The unifying theme of the books is the relevance and contributions of the field of human factors to design for an aging population.

Designing Training and Instructional Programs for Older Adults
Sara J. Czaja, Joseph Sharit

Designing Technology Training for Older Adults in Continuing Care Retirement Communities
Shelia R. Cotten, Elizabeth A. Yost, Ronald W. Berkowsky, Vicki Winstead, William A. Anderson

Designing for Older Adults
Principles and Creative Human Factors Approaches, Third Edition
Sara J. Czaja, Walter R. Boot, Neil Charness, Wendy A. Rogers

Designing Transportation Systems for Older Adults
Carryl L. Baldwin, Bridget A. Lewis, Pamela M. Greenwood

Designing Displays for Older Adults, Second Edition
Anne McLaughlin, Richard Pak

Designing for Older Adults: Case Studies, Methods, and Tools
Walter Boot, Neil Charness, Sara J Czaja, Wendy A. Rogers

Designing Robots to Improve Quality of Life for Older Adults
Wendy A. Rogers and Tracy L. Mitzner

For more information about this series, please visit: www.crcpress.com/Human-Factors-and-Aging-Series/book-series/CRCHUMFACAGI

Designing Robots to Improve Quality of Life for Older Adults

Wendy A. Rogers, Ph.D. and
Tracy L. Mitzner, Ph.D.

CRC Press
Taylor & Francis Group
Boca Raton London New York

CRC Press is an imprint of the
Taylor & Francis Group, an **informa** business

First edition published 2026
by CRC Press
2385 NW Executive Center Drive, Suite 320, Boca Raton FL 33431

and by CRC Press
4 Park Square, Milton Park, Abingdon, Oxon, OX14 4RN

CRC Press is an imprint of Taylor & Francis Group, LLC

ISBN: 9781032636825 (hbk)
ISBN: 9781032656632 (pbk)
ISBN: 9781032656649 (ebk)

DOI: 10.1201/9781032656649

Typeset in Palatino
by codeMantra

We dedicate this book to Dr. Cory-Ann Smarr Kane. She was an enthusiastic and creative researcher, and her contributions to the field of human–robot interaction are evidenced by our references to her work in this book. She was taken from us far too soon, but her memory and her influence live on.

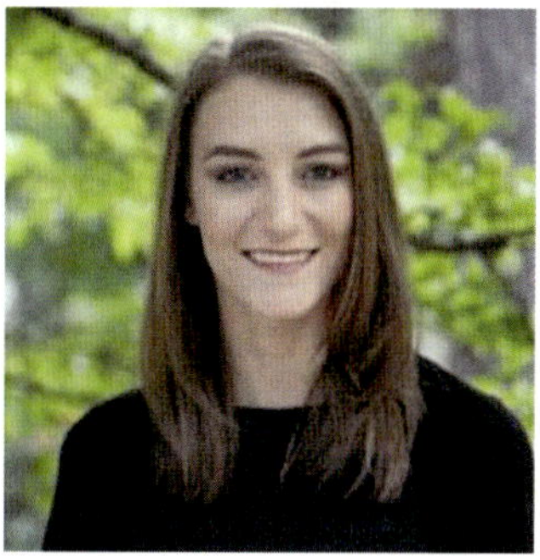

Contents

Foreword

Back in 2010, I had the good fortune of beginning a long and fruitful collaboration with Professor Wendy Rogers. At the time, we were both on the faculty at Georgia Tech. I was a junior faculty member focused on robots for healthcare, and she was a professor with deep expertise in technology for older adults. Though our backgrounds differed with me coming from the world of computer science and Professor Rogers coming from the world of psychology, we shared a practical mindset and a sincere passion for enabling robots to benefit older adults.

Together with Dr. Tracy Mitzner and others, we initially worked with a state-of-the-art mobile robot with two arms named the PR2 (Personal Robot 2) developed by Willow Garage. As one of the most exciting research robots at the time and weighing almost 500 pounds, the PR2 was both a metaphorical and literal giant in the field. Despite its size, the PR2 enabled our team to investigate interactions between robots and older adults and thereby gain insights grounded by real-world use.

Now, 14 years later, this iterative process of discovery continues. Dr. Aaron Edsinger and I lead Hello Robot, Inc., which we founded to commercialize Stretch, a modestly sized 54-pound mobile robot with an arm that is intended to enhance life for everyone, including older adults. Stretch's design directly benefited from Professor Rogers' guidance, and our collaboration described in Chapter 8 has led to surprising discoveries about how robots such as Stretch can benefit older adults in their homes.

Working with Professor Rogers changed the way I think about designing robots. While our collaborations have included a large number of people from diverse backgrounds, it is not realistic for everyone to collaborate with Professor Rogers! So, I am grateful that she and Dr. Mitzner have written *Designing Robots to Improve Quality of Life for Older Adults*. With this book, more people can learn useful ways of thinking about human-centric robot design and how to make progress toward real robots that improve quality of life for older adults.

Robots are still an emerging technology. Despite ambitious efforts by teams of talented and sincere individuals, robots have yet to live up to their potential. At the time of writing this foreword, most home robots that benefit older adults are specialized robots such as floor cleaners and pool cleaners. Yet, as Professor Rogers and Dr. Mitzner make clear, robots have remarkable potential, and the underlying technologies continue to improve.

Society is at the beginning of a long journey. So, you, dear reader, have an opportunity to influence the future. Will versatile home robots benefit millions of older adults in five years or five decades? Will robots meaningfully benefit older adults or inadvertently degrade quality of life? The answers to these questions and more depend on the actions we take today.

Whether you are just starting out or are already an expert, I am heartened that you are reading this book. I believe its guidance can help us create a more favorable future sooner. Farewell on your journey!

Charlie Kemp, Ph.D.
Co-founder of Hello Robot, Inc.

Preface

We first started conducting research on human–robot interaction (HRI) issues around 2007 at the Human Factors and Aging (HFA) Laboratory when it was located at the Georgia Institute of Technology, co-directed by Dr. Wendy A. Rogers and Dr. Arthur (Dan) Fisk, with Dr. Tracy L. Mitzner as its Associate Director. We were inspired by our collaborations with Dr. Charlie Kemp as well as interactions with Dr. Andrea Thomaz and Dr. Ayanna Howard, who were all faculty members at the time at Georgia Tech. Numerous graduate students in our lab were engaged in HRI research including Neta Ezer, Akanksha Prakash, Jenay Beer, Kathi Olson, and Cory-Ann Smarr. Our HRI research continued after the HFA Laboratory moved to the University of Illinois Urbana-Champaign in 2017 with Wendy Rogers and Person in Design was founded by Tracy Mitzner. Graduate student research (Megan Bayles) and postdoctoral fellows joining the lab continued to focus on this topic (Travis Kadylak, Samuel Olatunji, Pallabi Bhowmick).

We decided to collect our decades of knowledge on the topic and propose a book as part of the *Human Factors and Aging Series* published by CRC Press, edited by Wendy Rogers. We kicked off our effort with a reconnaissance trip to the CES Conference in Las Vegas, Nevada, in January 2023. We were inspired by the advanced robotic technologies being presented and the recognition by developers that older adults could benefit from their products. However, it was clear to us that an awareness of human factors processes, an understanding of older adults' needs and preferences, and a recognition of the complexity of HRI were going to have to be incorporated into the design process if these innovations were to be translated into improved quality of life for older adults.

That is the goal of this book: to provide a comprehensive state-of-the-science review of the topic of designing robots for older adults. We provide a framework for HRI that is specific to design of robots for older adults, including a focus on human, robot, interaction, and environment dimensions. This systematic approach is critical for the development of robots that will be adopted by older adults. We provide an overview of the fundamentals of aging that need to be considered when designing robots for older adults. We emphasize the heterogeneity of the older adult population and discuss demographic, perceptual, motor, and cognitive capabilities that might impact HRI. We provide an overview of different types of robots (e.g., humanoid, machinelike, pet-like). We explore the capabilities that robots might need to have. We identify the known facilitators and barriers for adoption, based on empirical literature. Moreover, we describe the potential of robots for different everyday activities including basic activities of daily living (ADLs), instrumental activities of daily living (IADLs), and enhanced activities of daily living (EADLs).

Numerous people in our professional and personal lives have supported our efforts to complete this book. We list them here, but this mention does not do justice to their contributions!

- Christy McGuire, *for editing, content, and general moral support!*
- Tongxin Sun, *for her creativity and the HRI framework design.*
- Henry Evans and Jane Evans, *for support of HRI research and willingness to share their stories and feedback on the draft.*
- Charlie Kemp, *for writing the foreword* and, along with his Hello Robot co-founder Aaron Edsinger, *for helping us learn about the complexities of starting a company to develop, produce, and market a robot that is designed to help people.*
- Samuel Olatunji, *for conceptual input and feedback on framework.*
- Vy Nguyen, *for insights and photography skills.*
- Cassie Payonk, *for background research and support with figures.*
- Members of the Human Factors and Aging Laboratory, *for feedback on the framework.*
- Jon Sanford, *for feedback on the framework.*
- Students in the HK 400 course "Human-Robot Interaction for Health & Wellness" and our older adult class panel, namely, Jim Fawcett, Kathleen Holden, Earl Kellogg, and Anna Merritt, *for insights on the content and reviews of early drafts of chapters.*
- CRC Press and our Editor James Hobbs, *for guidance and patience throughout the writing process.*
- Our families, *for their continued support and patience, especially Dan Fisk who also provided conceptual input along the way, and Jerry, Anders, and Lela Hart for their steadfast encouragement.*

We have dedicated this book to Dr. Cory-Ann Smarr Kane, who studied HRI as a graduate student – her early work was recognized in 2012 when she was the lead on the paper receiving the Human Factors and Ergonomics Society (HFES) Arnold M. Small Aging Technical Group Best Student Paper Award:

- Smarr, C.-A., Prakash, A., Beer, J. M., Mitzner, T. L., Kemp, C. C., & Rogers, W. A. (2012, October). *Older adults' preferences for and acceptance of robot assistance for everyday living tasks.* Presented at the Human Factors and Ergonomics Society 56th Annual Meeting, Boston, MA.

She conducted both her master's thesis and doctoral dissertation on HRI-related topics:

- Smarr, C.-A. (2011). *Emotion and motion: Age-related differences in recognizing virtual agent facial expressions.* Master's thesis, Georgia Institute of Technology, Atlanta, GA.
- Smarr, C.-A. (2014). *Applying a qualitative framework of acceptance of personal robots.* Doctoral dissertation, Georgia Institute of Technology, Atlanta, GA.

Cory was a creative and enthusiastic researcher; we know she would have been excited about having her work highlighted in this book. She believed in the potential of robots to provide support for everyday activities. Sadly, she was taken from the world at a young age, but she leaves a professional legacy of her work as well as a personal legacy of her two daughters to continue her memory.

This book is intended for a broad audience including gerontologists, human factors/ergonomics specialists, and the design community. We have translated the research on aging, human factors, and HRI into guidance for practitioners who design robots for a range of applications. We hope that the readers of this book are inspired to design robots that will improve quality of life for older adults.

– Wendy A. Rogers, Ph.D.
– Tracy L. Mitzner, Ph.D.

About the Authors

Wendy A. Rogers, Ph.D., is Khan Professor of Applied Health Sciences at the University of Illinois Urbana-Champaign. She received her B.A. from the University of Massachusetts-Dartmouth, and her M.S. and Ph.D. from the Georgia Institute of Technology. She is a Certified Human Factors Professional (BCPE Certificate #1539). Her research focuses on advanced technology design to support autonomy of older adults with and without disabilities. She explores the benefits of technologies including robots, smart home technology, digital health, wearables, and telehealth for cognitive, physical, and emotional health. She is the Director of the McKechnie Family LIFE Home and the Human Factors and Aging Laboratory, and the Program Director of CHART (Collaborations in Health, Aging, Research, and Technology). She is funded by the National Institutes of Health through the National Institute on Aging as part of the *Center for Research and Education on Aging and Technology Enhancement* (CREATE), the National Institute of Nursing Research, and the Department of Health and Human Services through the National Institute on Disability, Independent Living, and Rehabilitation Research through Rehabilitation Engineering Research Centers on *Technologies to Support Aging-in-Place for People with Long-Term Disabilities* (TechSAge) and *Center for Enhancing Neurocognitive Health, Abilities, Networks, and Community Engagement* (ENHANCE).

Tracy L. Mitzner, Ph.D., is the founder and Principal Research Scientist at Person in Design, a consulting firm specializing in leveraging scientific research to drive technology design for older adults, including those with disabilities. She received her B.A. from Beloit College and her M.A., Ph.D., and Certificate in Gerontology from the University of Kansas. She completed a postdoctoral fellowship in Cognitive Aging at the Georgia Institute of Technology. She continued her career at Georgia Tech as a Research Scientist for 22 years, including time in the School of Psychology and the Center for Inclusive Design and Innovation. Dr. Mitzner's research interests include the design of emerging technologies (mobile applications, health monitoring, telepresence, robotics), particularly for applications to facilitate social and physical wellness. She is funded by the National Institutes of Health through the National Institute on Aging as part of the CREATE and the Department of Health and Human Services through the National Institute on Disability, Independent Living, and Rehabilitation Research through Rehabilitation Engineering Research Center on *Technologies to Support Aging-in-Place for People with Long-Term Disabilities* (TechSAge).

1

Introduction and overview

1.1 Potential of robots to support older adults

The title of this book is *Designing Robots to Improve Quality of Life for Older Adults*. Presumably, then, robots have the potential to do so. However, we know that robots are not yet ubiquitous in our daily lives and that the typical older adult likely does not have a robot assisting them with everyday activities.

Adults over age 60 or 65 comprise a major proportion of the population in the United States as well as globally. Older adults have been found to be quite open to the idea of interacting with robots, although they have preferences for the nature of the tasks that they want the robot to do for/with them as well as what they want the robot to look like. These preferences are not set in stone but should be considered in the process of design and deployment. Moreover, it is crucial to involve older adults throughout the design process from formative to summative evaluation and even beyond to the integration of the robot into their everyday activities. The extant research provides valuable guidance regarding the capabilities and limitations of older adults that might influence their ability to interact with a personal robot. Additionally, much is known about the needs of older adults that might be met by a robot. Our goal in this book is to provide a framework that can be used to guide the development of robots that will be useful to and usable by older adults.

1.2 Media representation vs. current state of science

For decades, robots have been depicted interacting with humans in news articles, popular press books, television shows, and movies. Sometimes they are helpful robots, supporting the needs of people as in the television series *The Jetsons*, wherein Rosey the Robot was the servant for the family catering to the needs and wants of the parents and children. In other cases, the robots are vengeful and menacing, as in *The Terminator* movie series. And there are many robots in between these extremes. Not only have the physical appearances of robots changed over time, but their capabilities in the media have changed as well. Figure 1.1 shows a timeline of media representation from 1927 to 2004.

DOI: 10.1201/9781032656649-1

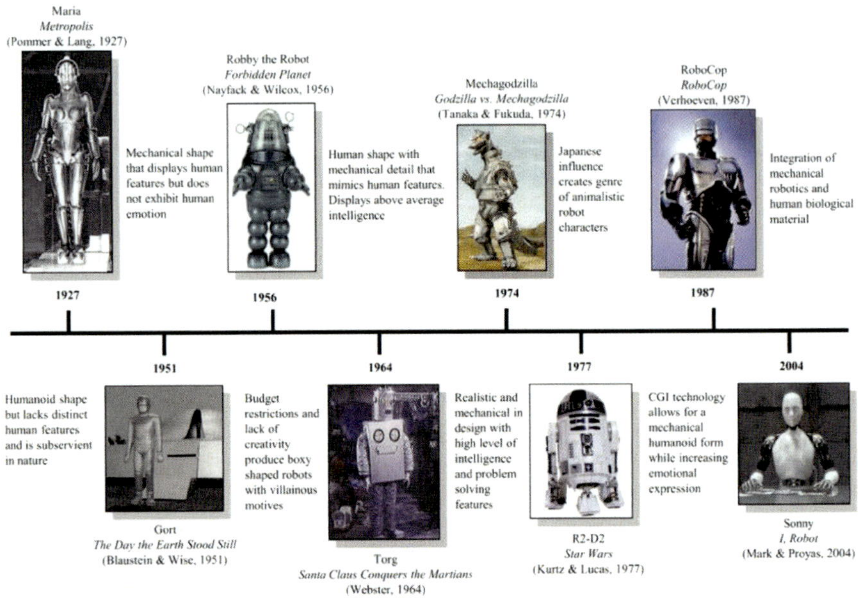

FIGURE 1.1
Robot trends in media (from: Schaefer et al., 2015).

These media representations typically do not reflect reality. Oftentimes the robots depicted have capabilities that are beyond what is technically possible, which will influence people's expectations of what a robot should be able to do. Incorrect expectations can affect adoption in different ways. For example, if a robot being introduced to older adults is less capable than expected, people may be impatient or frustrated in their interactions. In addition, the user may think that the robot is able to do more than it actually can do, resulting in overreliance or misplaced trust.

More recently, and with specific relevance to older adults, high-profile stories about how robots can or should or should not be used to support older adults can influence attitudes of older adults as well as their family members and professional caregivers. The titles of a few recent examples are telling, in terms of the potential hype or bias either in favor of or against robots. In addition, the stories tend to be very ageist in their depiction of older adults, with little respect for them as people or awareness of their diversity of capabilities and needs.

- "For older people who are lonely, is the solution a robot friend?" (*New York Times*, July 6, 2024)
- "Senior citizens are getting robotic pets to combat loneliness: 'There's somebody here listening to me' Animatronic stuffed animals are providing 'companionship' to the elderly" (*People Magazine*, June 17, 2024)
- "This robot catches grandma before she falls" (*Washington Post*, September 10, 2022)

- "These robots may soon help us care for our older relatives" (*USA Today*, December 19, 2019)
- "Should you leave grandma with the robot?" (*NPR*, October 6, 2017)

Advancements in technology are rapid in terms of sensors, artificial intelligence, hardware, and so on. But how do we enable the design of robots to achieve what is represented in the media and that the potential is met, is accessible, and represents reality for a person in their daily life? A guiding principle of this book is to provide background knowledge and design approaches that can enable the future to meet the present media representations. And, of course, we mean the *positive* media representations wherein the robot is supporting the needs of older adults.

1.3 What is a robot?

Defining what we mean by a robot may be more complicated than one might imagine. People have an image of robots, often influenced by media depictions. Robot developers might have specific components in mind when they think about a robot. Companies might market a product as a robot to enhance market share. As a starting point, we have traced the history of robot definitions, a sampling of which is provided in Figure 1.2.

As is evident, there is not a consensus on how to define a robot. We adopt a very broad definition for this book. A robot has a physical embodiment that can sense, plan, and act on the environment. The physical embodiment can vary

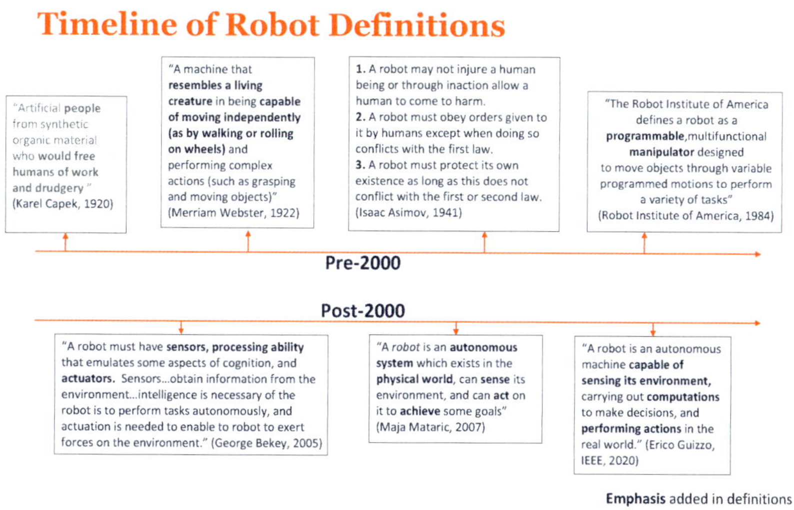

FIGURE 1.2
Timeline of robot definitions.

widely, as will become clear from our examples. How it senses and plans is not our focus – rather we will explore what it needs to sense and plan to effectively support the needs of older adults. Likewise, the specifics of how it acts on the environment is going to be dependent on what the robot needs to do.

1.4 Categories of robots

Robots come in all shapes and sizes and are not easily categorized as they may have multiple functions and features. Moreover, many robots are not relevant to older adults, such as agricultural robots, construction robots, industrial robots, logistic robots, medical robots, military robots, and search-and-rescue robots, among others. We will focus on the broad categories of robots that are most relevant to older adults and their everyday activities.

- An *assistive robot* can be broadly defined as a robot that gives aid to a human user. That might mean that the robot is performing a task for the person, or it may assist the human in performing the task by making it easier.
- *Educational robots* assist students in learning new things. Although often targeted to children, educational robots could support learning new skills or rehabilitation exercises, or other activities for people of all ages.
- *Exoskeleton robots* are wearable robots that can be used for rehabilitation purposes to assist with therapy or to support mobility.
- *Manipulator robots* are outfitted with some type of end effector that can interact with objects in the environment. It might be a gripper, a hand, a tow-hook, or a shovel – it can be any type of extension that enables the robot to manipulate an item.
- *Mobile robots* can move about in a physical space. Their mobility may be instantiated with wheels, tracks, legs, rollerballs, or any variety of mechanism.
- *Service robots* perform specific tasks such as cleaning (e.g., vacuuming, pool cleaning, sanitation), mowing, or security patrolling.
- *Social robots* are those that provide or assist with social interaction or emotional support. Social interaction can consist of holding a conversation, playing games, or providing emotional engagement, any of which can be verbal or non-verbal. Social intelligence in this context can span from responding to touch to being able to detect emotion from facial expression.
- *Telepresence robots* enable people to remotely participate in an event through video, often with the ability to move around a space. A telepresence robot is sometimes described as a "videochat platform on wheels."

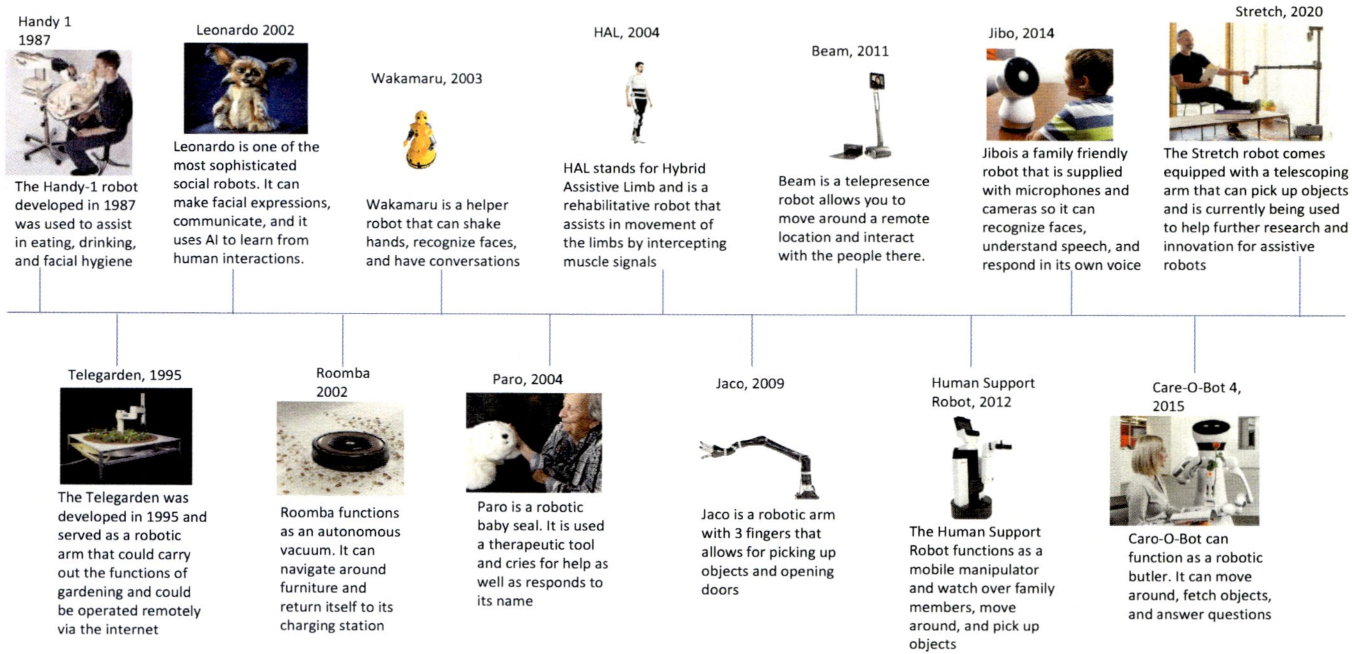

FIGURE 1.3
Timeline of assistive robots (adapted from: Balaguer et al., 2003 and https://robotsguide.com/robots).

These categories are not mutually exclusive. As will be evident from the examples provided throughout the book, robots often fit into multiple categories. A robot may be a "mobile manipulator" and a "socially assistive" robot for instance. Note that the categorization is about the functionality of the robot and what it is intended to do. Underlying all these categories is the vast programming and intelligence required to accomplish these functions. Given that this is not an engineering-focused book, we do not describe the technical components of robots but instead explore the use of robots from the perspective of the human.

In addition to growth in the breadth of robot categories, robots within categories have evolved tremendously over time. For example, Figure 1.3 provides examples of assistive robots and how they have changed from 1987 to 2020. Yet despite these robots being developed and touted as useful for older adults, few of them are available today for personal use in the homes of older adults.

1.5 Human–robot interaction framework

Human–robot interaction (HRI), by definition, encompasses the human, the robot, and their interaction. The interaction has the goal of performing a task together, and it occurs within a broader context. We developed the HRI framework illustrated in Figure 1.4 to specify these different components, along with exemplars of each (see Rogers & Mitzner, 2017, for an earlier version

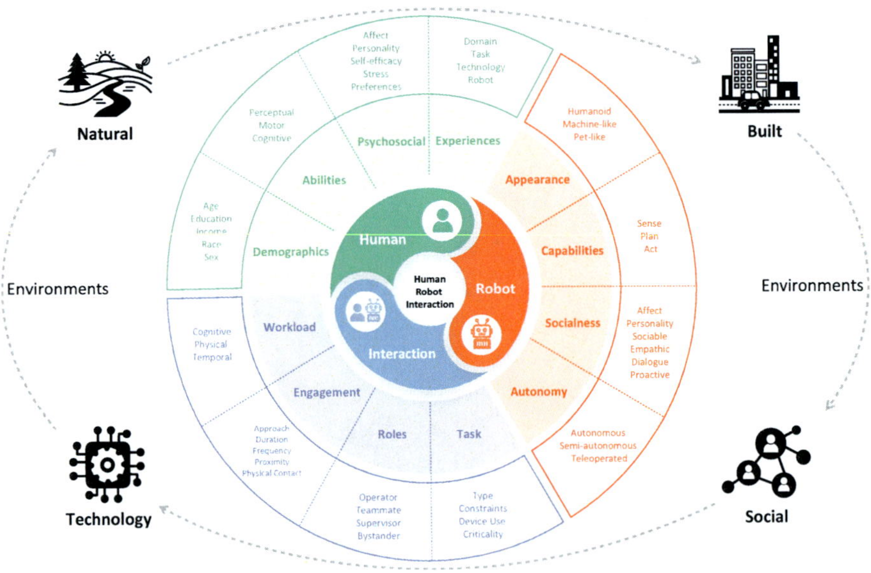

FIGURE 1.4
HRI framework.

of this framework). The framework is based on user-centered and universal design principles that encompass the four primary dimensions of HRI: the *human*, the *robot*, the *interaction*, and the *environment*. These dimensions represent the breadth of variables that should be considered in the design of a robot and the many factors that impact HRI. The framework can be used by robot developers to guide design priorities and specifications, as well as by researchers to delineate factors that may influence HRI. It will also serve as the underlying organization for this book. We describe each dimension here briefly with each receiving an in-depth treatment in subsequent chapters.

The human dimension consists of characteristics such as demographics, abilities, psychosocial attributes, and experiences. Demographic variables include age, education, income, race, and sex. In this book, we explore in depth the varied ways HRI may be influenced by age, specifically by being an older adult. One's age will impact needs and preferences for robot design. Abilities such as perceptual, motor, and cognitive are highlighted given the expansive literature on age-related changes on these abilities. Psychosocial variables such as affect, personality, self-efficacy, stress, and preferences can also influence HRI. Lastly, a person's experiences regarding different domains, tasks, technologies, and robots will impact HRI.

The robot dimension of our framework includes characteristics such as appearance, capabilities, socialness, and autonomy. A robot's appearance can generally be categorized as humanoid, machinelike, or pet-like. A robot's capabilities include the ability to sense, plan, and act. Socialness variables include affect, personality, sociability, empathy, dialogue, and proactiveness. The robot can be fully autonomous, semiautonomous, or teleoperated.

The interaction dimension reflects the task, interaction roles, engagement, and workload components. The task characteristics include type, constraints, device use, and criticality. Roles refer to how a person participates in the interaction as an operator, teammate, supervisor, or bystander. Engagement includes the approach, duration, frequency, proximity, and physical contact required for the interaction. Lastly, workload refers to the cognitive, physical, and/or temporal work demands that the interaction requires.

The environment dimension refers to the natural, built, social, and technology environments in which the HRI takes place. The natural environment includes land, water, air, plants, climate, and animals. The built environment refers to the human-made aspects of the environment such as homes, buildings, streets, open spaces, and infrastructure. The social environment refers to other people such as family, friends, co-workers, care network, and other service providers. The technology environment represents the idea of a technology ecology that might include the robot, smart technologies, digital home assistant, and appliances.

Our HRI framework is meant to be broad and guiding; it is neither comprehensive nor exhaustive. The topics provided are only representative examples. The exact characteristics that would be relevant for a particular human, robot, interaction, and environment will vary and may only include some of the examples presented in the framework. For the purposes of this book, we will highlight characteristics that are especially relevant for the use case of designing robots for older adults. Throughout this book, we will refer to this framework to highlight design considerations for designing robots to support the quality of life for older adults.

1.6 Goals for this book

Our goal for this book is to provide a state-of-the-science review of the topic of designing robots for older adults. Our HRI framework is specific to design of robots for older adults and serves as a starting point for the development of a robot or the selection of an existing robot for use by older adults. In either case, there is a process that should be followed: namely, to consider the different dimensions and use this information to guide the design and deployment process. Who will be using the robot? What are their needs and how might the robot meet these needs? What task(s) will be performed by the human and the robot? What is the interaction context – indoors/outdoors, multiple people in the area, or need for integration with other technology? Asking these questions and considering the complexity of the HRI context will provide valuable direction for the developer.

This systematic approach is critical for the development of robots that will be adopted by older adults. In Chapter 2, we focus on the human characteristics, providing an overview of the fundamentals of aging that need to be considered when designing robots for older adults. We emphasize the heterogeneity of the older adult population and discuss demographic, perceptual, motor, and cognitive capabilities that might impact HRI. Chapter 3 focuses on the robot characteristics: what they look like, what they can do, and how social or autonomous they are. Chapter 4 is about the interaction itself. What is it that the robot and the human are trying to accomplish? As such, we discuss tasks, roles, the nature of the engagement, and the workload imposed on the human user. Chapter 5 explores the influence of different interaction environments. Where will the robot be used and how might that environment influence design decisions? Chapter 6 considers the myriad ethical issues that designers must be aware of. Ethical considerations such as privacy, safety, and reliance are integral to the design process and must be considered from conception to implementation. Each of these chapters concludes with *Design Guidelines*. Our goal is to provide actionable guidance that can increase the likelihood that a robot will be appropriately designed to meet the needs of the users, to achieve their goals, and with consideration for the context of use.

Chapter 7 delves into design methods and assessment measures that are relevant to HRI. We provide an overview of user-centered design methods and guidance for appropriate measures for acceptance, reliance, trust, preferences, usability, and so on.

In Chapter 8, we illustrate the application of the HRI framework. We provide details of a cross-cutting case study that draws from several years of our own research to show how the dimensions of the framework relate to the iterative design of a specific robot. Throughout, we emphasize the need to follow fundamental human factors processes and participatory design approaches that engage older adults in the design process.

In Chapter 9, we discuss implementation considerations. Even if the systematic design process has been followed, the ultimate test is the degree to which there is uptake of the robot in people's lives. We present models of technology adoption, diffusion of innovations, and technology acceptance. In addition, we consider the importance of maintenance – if robots will be in homes and public spaces, how do we ensure they remain functional? What happens if they break down?

Chapter 10 provides concluding remarks that revisit the potential for robots and the importance of user-centered design. We review the guidelines and lessons learned presented in individual chapters to provide a roadmap for successful robot design.

At the end of each chapter, we provide a set of recommended readings and links. These are intended to provide the interested reader with direction for exploring topics in the chapter in more depth.

The book is intended for a broad audience including engineers, designers, gerontologists, architects, healthcare providers, and policymakers. Our goal is to translate research on aging, human factors, and HRI into guidance that will be usable for practitioners who design or deploy robots for a range of applications. In addition, we hope to provide a resource for students who are learning about human factors, design for aging, and HRI. Together, we can advance design and deployment of robots to achieve the lofty goal of our title: *Designing Robots to Improve Quality of Life for Older Adults.*

Recommended readings and links

Readings

Beer, J. M., Prakash, A., Smarr, C.-A., Chen, T. L., Hawkins, K., Nguyen, H., Deyle, T., Mitzner, T. L., Kemp, C. C., & Rogers, W. A. (2017). Older users' acceptance of an assistive robot: Attitudinal changes following brief exposure. *Gerontechnology, 16*(1), 21–36. https://doi.org/10.4017/gt.2017.16.1.003.00

Gasteiger, N., Loveys, K., Law, M., & Broadbent, E. (2021). Friends from the future: A scoping review of research into robots and computer agents to combat loneliness in older people. *Clinical Interventions in Aging, 16,* 941–971. https://doi.org/10.2147/cia.s282709

Schaefer, K. E., Adams, J. K., Cook, J. G., Bardwell-Owens, A., & Hancock, P. A. (2015). The future of robotic design: Trends from the history of media representations. *Ergonomics in Design, 23*(1), 13–19. https://doi.org/10.1177/1064804614562214

Stuck, R. E., & Rogers, W. A. (2018). Older adults' perceptions of supporting factors of trust in a robot care provider. *Journal of Robotics, 2018,* 1–11. https://doi.org/10.1155/2018/6519713

Wiczorek, R., Bayles, M. A., & Rogers, W. A. (2020). Domestic robots for older adults: Design approaches and recommendations. In L. Moody, A. Woodcock, D. McDonagh, & L. C. Jain (Eds.), *Design of assistive technology for ageing populations* (pp. 203–219). Springer. https://doi.org/10.1007/978-3-030-26292-1_11

Links

Robots for humanity:
https://r4h.org/

Robots guide:
https://robotsguide.com/robots

The Jetsons:
https://www.imdb.com/title/tt0055683/

The Terminator series:
https://www.imdb.com/list/ls073555125/

2

Human characteristics

2.1 Overview of human characteristics

One key component of our human–robot interaction (HRI) framework is human characteristics (see Figure 2.1). In this book, we focus on the case when the human interacting with the robot is an older adult. Older adulthood is generally considered as 60 and older according to the World Health Organization. However, in the United States, 65 years often defines older adulthood given this has historically been retirement age. However, within the workforce, 40 years of age and older often defines an older worker. Hence, the exact age used to define an older person can vary given the context. For this book, reference to an older person will typically mean age 65+.

By 2050, the world population age 65 and older is estimated to reach 1.6 billion, more than twice as many people as in 2021, meaning that one in six people will be 65 and older (see Figure 2.2). With this population shift comes a large set of health, social, and economic challenges.

Interest is growing in understanding how robots may be able to support the increasing population of older adults, as it is projected to exceed the caregiving workforce. There is additional value in designing robots to support older adults in that most prefer to remain in their home and community of choice. Maintaining control over the decisions that impact their daily lives can lead to higher quality of life and lower mortality rates. Robot assistance could extend the time in which older adults retain their autonomy.

When designing robots, it is imperative to consider the characteristics of the human user including demographics, abilities, psychosocial, and experiences. These categories are not exhaustive, and each one can influence the acceptance or use of a robot in multiple ways. Age-associated characteristics relate to specific needs and preferences for robotic support, as well as their ability to use a robot given that older adults tend to have less technology experience than younger adults. Moreover, with age comes an increased need for support for a wide variety of tasks, which is discussed in detail in Chapter 4. As the number of older adults in society is increasing exponentially, robot

DOI: 10.1201/9781032656649-2

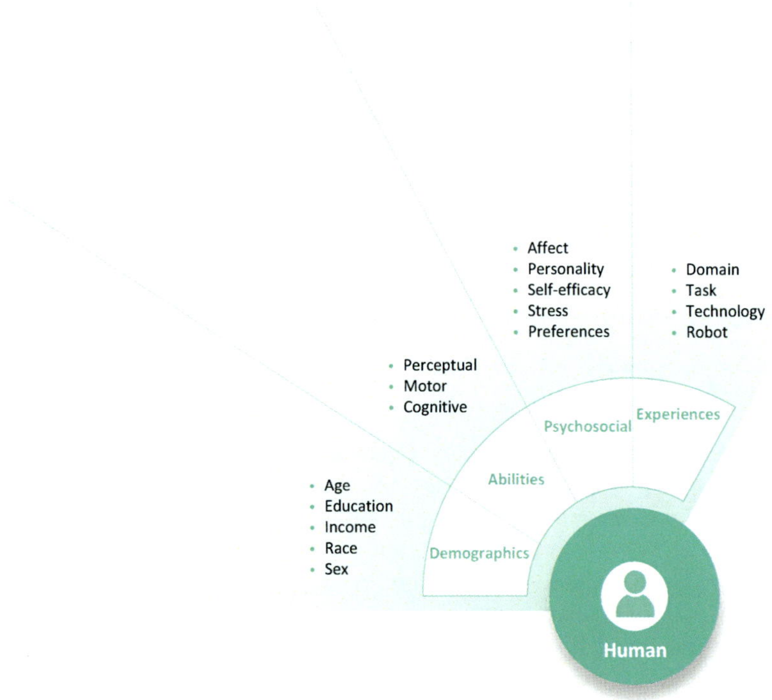

FIGURE 2.1
HRI framework: human characteristics.

developers have the opportunity to address the accompanying needs for support and care, thereby supporting older adults' independence and quality of life.

Older adults' characteristics, daily experiences, and perspectives are unique from other age groups. Within the older adult population, there is great variability as well. Differences in race, education, and income impact lifestyle factors and access to healthcare, which can create large disparities in health status and functional abilities. Experiences accumulated over one's younger life can influence psychological status and well-being in older adulthood. Moreover, there can be wide variability in social relationships and support networks in older age devoid of the built-in social environments provided by school and work. Our HRI framework reflects how variability in human characteristics such as demographics, psychosocial abilities, and experiences should be considered in the design of robots. Below we describe these characteristics in the context of older adults.

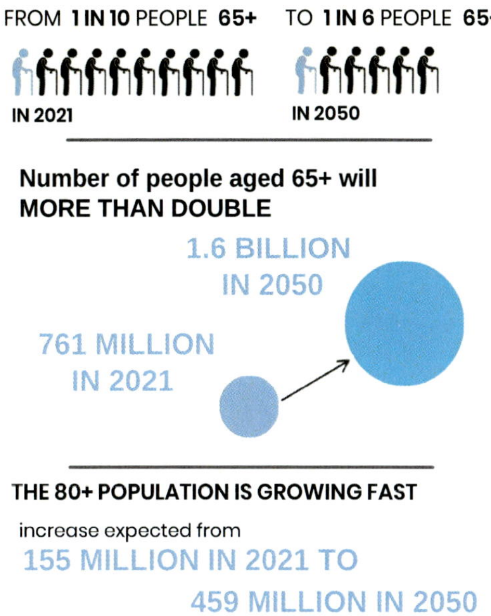

FIGURE 2.2
Estimated growth of population aged 65+ and 80+ from 2021 to 2050 (adapted from: UN DESA, 2023).

2.2 Demographics

Demographics, such an individual's age, education, income, race, and sex, can impact HRI in a variety of ways. As mentioned, the age range of older adulthood is commonly considered to be 65 years of age and over, but even within the population of older adults, age itself is still an important consideration for HRI. The needs and preferences for robotic support by a 65-year-old are likely quite different from those of a 95-year-old. For example, a 95-year-old is more likely to experience strength and mobility limitations, cognitive declines, and increased needs for support with everyday tasks. With age comes increased risk for more complex healthcare needs including chronic conditions, comorbidities, and mental health conditions (Figure 2.3).

Many demographic characteristics are interrelated; for example, education and income are closely connected to other human characteristics. Lower education is correlated with lower income, as well as lower cognitive function in older age and less technology experience. Hence, if one were to design a robot with the input of only highly educated older adults, the robot may not be usable by the larger older adult population. Demographic characteristics can influence the social environment (see Chapter 5). Race plays a key factor

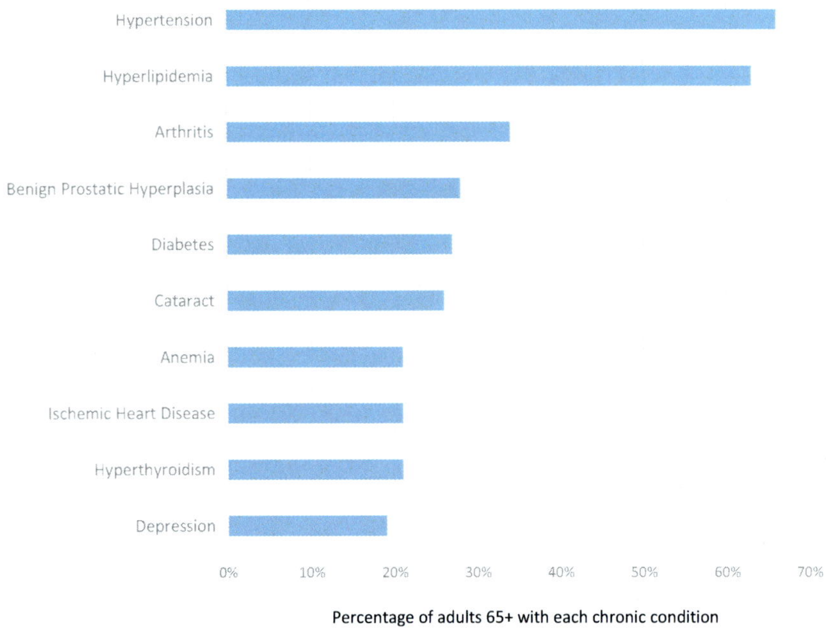

FIGURE 2.3
Ten most common chronic conditions for adults aged 65+ (from: Centers for Medicare & Medicaid Services, 2021).

in both education and income, given social history such as redlining, forced integration, and exclusionary banking practices. In addition, ethnicity can be associated with cultural norms regarding attitudes about aging, caring for older family members, and intergenerational living expectations. Similarly, sex is associated with norms about household activities and caregiving that can impact preferences for and acceptance of robotic support.

2.3 Abilities

A wide range of perceptual, motor, and cognitive abilities decline with age (for a review, see Czaja et al., 2019). Robot support may compensate for some of these declines to maximize an older adult's independence and autonomy.

2.3.1 Perceptual

Age-related vision declines include decreased visual acuity, reduced contrast sensitivity, increased sensitivity to glare, and increased prevalence of cataracts, glaucoma, and age-related macular degeneration. These declines can begin to impact one's everyday life as early as 40 years of age and can be exacerbated by chronic conditions such as diabetes and high blood pressure. Robots have the potential to produce additional lighting, convert text to voice, enlarge text, or provide alerts about obstacles.

Hearing declines include presbycusis (age-related hearing loss, especially for high-frequency sounds) and reduced ability to hear in noisy environments, such as situations with background noise. These declines can also begin as early as middle age. Robots could provide closed captioning or other accommodations in these environments.

Compensation for age-related declines in taste, smell, and touch sensitivity could also be provided by robots. For example, robots could provide a safety value by alerting an older person of the presence of smoke before the person could detect it or that a food has spoiled before they eat it. With awareness of these sensory declines, robots could incorporate sensors that compensate and provide augmented information about the environment.

2.3.2 Motor

Motor abilities that decline with age include strength, speed, coordination, balance, reaction time, and learning. These declines can accelerate later in older adulthood (after age 75). The most significant impact of these declines is an increase in fall risk. Falls are a leading cause of death in people over 65. Alternatively, they can cause hip fractures that typically require hospitalization and may take a significant amount of time to heal and recover from. Along with vision declines, motor declines can also impede one's ability to safely control a car. Robotic cars and mobility support devices hold much promise for reducing accident and fall risk. Robotic devices could assess homes and community spaces for fall risks and recommend modifications, as well as provide support in the event of a fall (e.g., notify family or emergency services).

2.3.3 Cognitive

Age-related cognitive changes include memory, processing speed, attention, executive function, language, and spatial declines. Cognitive declines may begin in middle age, but most do not impact everyday life until later ages, such as after 70. Cognitive impairment increases with age as well, including mild cognitive impairment (MCI) and various types of dementia (e.g., Alzheimer's, Lewy body, vascular). Robotic support for these declines could include providing alerts and alarms for important events (e.g., healthcare appointments, birthdays) and providing support for activities that place heavy demands on memory (e.g., navigating unfamiliar places, processing new healthcare information, learning new skills).

Some cognitive abilities are stable or can increase with age, such as vocabulary and world knowledge. Robots should be designed to reflect the wisdom older adults have accumulated. It is critical that robots are respectful and avoid being patronizing or using elderspeak. Elderspeak is a communication style that involves speaking to older adults in a way that is perceived as condescending and demoralizing. It can include simplified vocabulary, slow and loud speech, "baby talk," use of diminutives, and over-explanation. Not only is it perceived negatively, but it is correlated with decreased self-esteem, increased feelings of dependency, and increased social withdrawal.

2.3.4 Disabilities

As more people are living longer, so is the population with newly acquired and long-term disabilities. The most common disability among older adults is mobility disability (walking or climbing steps), followed by hearing, independent living, cognitive (remembering and concentrating), self-care, and vision disabilities, respectively (Figure 2.4). Robots could provide assistance in performing activities that are difficult for this population, such as reaching for items that are too high or too low, answering the front door, facilitating showering/bathing, or ensuring the home is secure after they have gone to bed. Moreover, robots could provide wayfinding support for

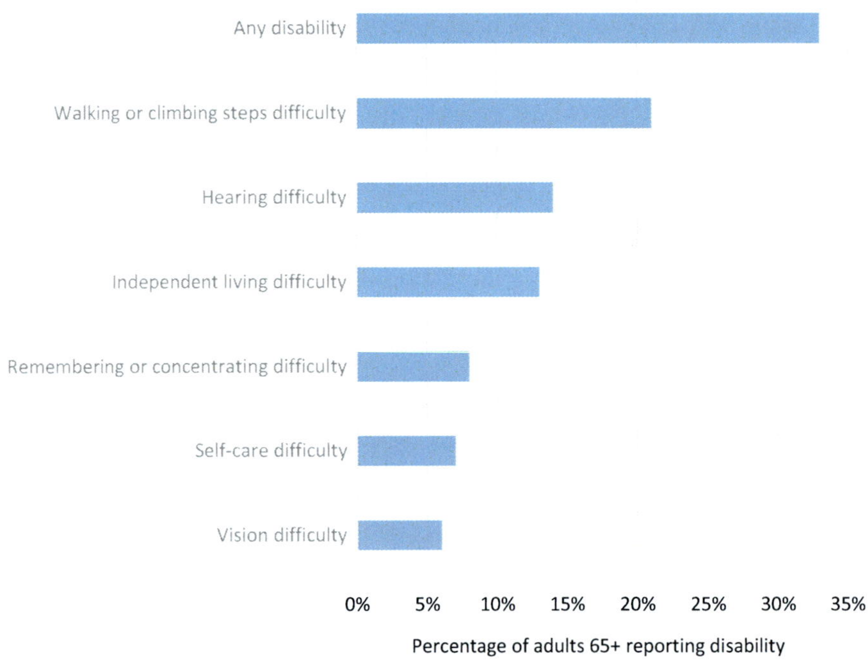

FIGURE 2.4
Prevalence of disabilities in older adults aged 65+ (adapted from: U.S. Administration for Community Living, 2023).

those aging with vision disabilities through support for navigation through environments. Robots could provide American Sign Language interpreting or voice to text for those who are Deaf or hard of hearing.

Robots have the potential to provide compensation for many age-related declines in abilities, but they need to be designed with older adult users in mind. Robot interfaces must be designed with consideration for age-related declines in perceptual, motor, and cognitive abilities. For example, any interface text or symbols should be of an appropriate size and contrast and consider lighting and potential for glare in the environment. Robot sounds should avoid high frequencies and consider any use of the robot where there may be significant background noise. Training and use need to take into account age-related declines in memory and provide appropriate support such as manuals and troubleshooting instructions (see recommended reading, Czaja & Sharit, 2012).

2.4 Psychosocial

Psychosocial characteristics such as affect, personality, self-efficacy, stress, and preferences have been explored regarding their influence on HRI for older adults. There are individual differences in affect and affective responses that can be influenced by many factors including genetics, personality characteristics, and earlier life experiences.

2.4.1 Affect

Affect refers broadly to emotional experiences or expressions, and within an individual, there is variability in affect. Moreover, affect and affective responses can vary from day to day and moment to moment. Many of those changes can be in reaction to life experiences, such as excitement for a family visitor or sadness about the loss of a friend. Changes in affect in the absence of an environmental cause could be indicative of a physical or neurological issue, or a reaction to a medication. Robots could be well suited for learning an individual's patterns of affect, providing intervention as needed. For negative affect in the normal range for that individual, the robot could recommend a self-soothing activity such as reading a book, going for a walk, or meditating. For negative or positive affect outside of the normal range for that individual, the robot could suggest the individual seek medical evaluation or notify a care partner.

Many age-related changes in affect are positive and adaptive in nature. For example, older adults tend to be better at regulating their emotions and have higher levels of positive affect, decreased reactivity to everyday stressors, and greater emotional complexity. Nevertheless, if these changes are not considered in HRI, a robot could be designed in a way in which it reacts inappropriately or misinterprets an older adult's response. If age-related changes in affect are taken into consideration, robots have the potential to detect and respond to complex emotional expression. They may be able to provide passive or active psychosocial assessments and indicate depression, pain, or discomfort as well.

One's affect can also influence how they perceive and interact with a robot. Positive affect, such as enjoyment, can enhance a user's acceptance and adoption of a robot. Alternatively, negative affect, such as frustration, can be a barrier to acceptance and adoption. Similarly, more positive emotional interactions could facilitate trust and reliance with a robot, and more negative emotional interactions could degrade trust and reliance. In these ways, a person's experience with technology, which we will discuss later, can create a cyclical effect wherein one negative experience could trigger a negative attitude about robots that perpetuates future negative attitudes and lack of acceptance and adoption. Thus, effective training and support is critical when learning how to use and interact robots (see Chapter 9 for more discussion of training considerations).

2.4.2 Personality

Personality refers to the persistent characteristics and behaviors of a person as they uniquely respond to life's experiences and circumstances. Personality, therefore, by definition, tends to be relatively stable with age. One of the most common personality models suggests five dimensions of personality:

- Openness to experience – intellectual curiosity, creativity, imagination
- Conscientiousness – organization, productiveness, responsibility
- Extraversion – sociability, assertiveness
- Agreeableness – compassion, respectfulness, trust in others
- Neuroticism – anxiety and depression tendencies

A robot could potentially collect observational or questionnaire data to determine where an individual's personality falls on these five dimensions. A robot could use any knowledge they have about an individual's personality to better predict their attitudes, preferences, and behavior. For instance, if an individual scores low on agreeableness, the robot might be able to facilitate trust in a new relationship, perhaps providing background information about the expertise, experience, and ratings of a new healthcare provider. There is some evidence of increased emotional stability in older adults, which corresponds with age-related increases in emotion regulation and decreases in reactivity to everyday stressors. Interestingly, those who score higher on the personality characteristics agreeableness and openness to experience have been shown to be more likely to accept technologies such as computers and smartphones; a similar pattern would be expected for robots.

2.4.3 Self-Efficacy

Self-efficacy is an individual's belief or confidence in their ability to complete a task or achieve a goal. It can be measured in a general sense or with respect to a certain behavior (e.g., exercise) or activity (e.g., using a technology). Self-efficacy can impact physical and mental health, as well as overall quality of life. If an older adult has high self-efficacy, they are more likely to engage in healthy behaviors, such as eating healthfully and exercising, and will, therefore, be more likely to have better health outcomes. Those with high self-efficacy are also more likely to have lower levels of depression and anxiety, and more likely to experience resilience in the midst of significant life stressors and transitions (e.g., retirement, moving homes, financial challenges, death of loved one). Self-efficacy is malleable and can benefit from interventions such as improved social support, therapy, or training. Robots could help to identify needs for improvement in self-efficacy and could identify (or possibly provide) necessary training and interventions.

Older adults with higher self-efficacy are more likely to use computers, the internet, and smartphones. Those with higher self-efficacy probably have more confidence to initiate using a new technology, seek help and support, and are more likely to persist and troubleshoot through challenges; they would thus be expected to make fewer negative internal attributions about mistakes in interacting with a robot. There is limited research on the interaction of aging, self-efficacy, and HRI, but it would be expected that people with higher self-efficacy about interacting with robots would have a more positive experiences learning to use robots and interacting with them. Positive early experiences with robots can potentially improve a person's self-efficacy for interacting with robots. Appropriate training and support when learning to use robots could therefore facilitate adoption of robots, perhaps by providing additional support for individuals with low self-efficacy.

2.4.4 Stress

Stress refers to emotional pressure or tension experienced by an individual. Common major stressors for older adults include retirement, moving homes, social isolation, physical and cognitive health challenges, financial concerns, and caring for or death of a loved one. Everyday stressors can include needing and finding assistance for activities, and transportation challenges. Learning to use a robot could induce stress for an older adult, given they tend to have less technology experience compared to younger adults.

High-stress personal situations (e.g., emergency alerting) have been highlighted as use cases for social robots for older adults. High stress is associated with users being less accurate at detecting automation errors (for both younger and older adults), which could impact HRI. There are also use cases in which robots provide comfort and companionship for older adults. Such an application could be impactful for the many older adults who live alone and are at a risk of social isolation. Social isolation is critical to address, given that it is associated with poor health outcomes and increased mortality risk. Some findings suggest that social robots may reduce stress for older adults, as measured by pulse rate, pulse oximetry, galvanic skin response, and saliva cortisol. There is evidence that robots can reduce stress for older adults with dementia.

2.4.5 Preferences

Technology preferences is another characteristic of an older adult robot user that can impact acceptance and adoption rates. People have preferences for how robots look (https://phys.org/news/2013) and how they behave. Some prefer robots that look more humanoid or familiar, whereas others prefer robots that look futuristic or non-humanoid, and those appearance preferences can be task-specific. They also have preferences for what they want the robot to assist with.

Our research has examined older adults' as well as professional care providers' preferences for robotic support for a variety of tasks. For example, the data in Figure 2.5 show the results from our study with older

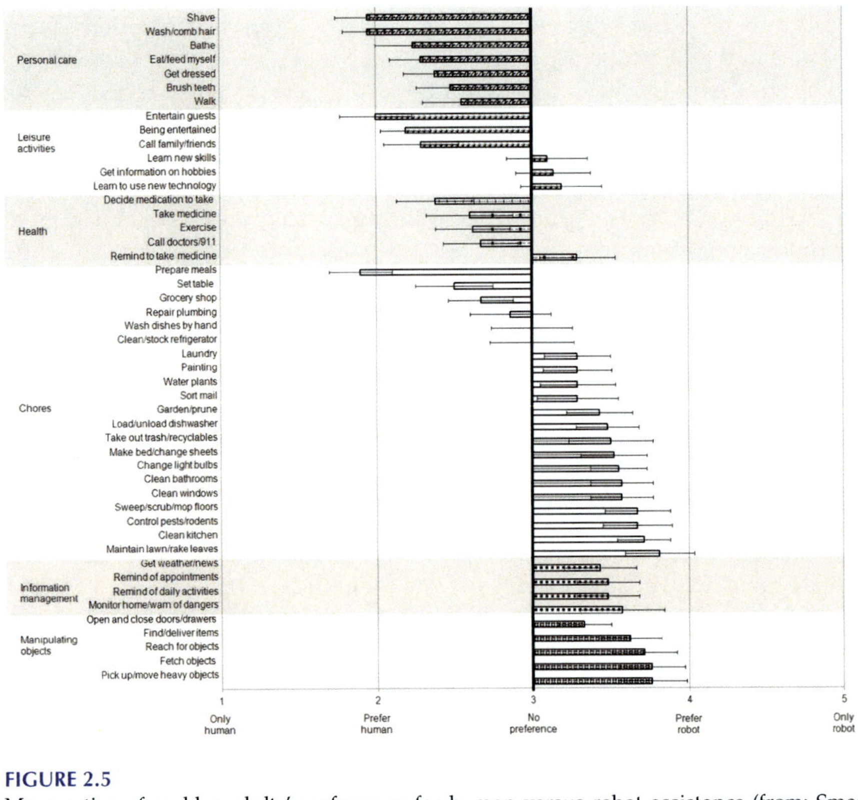

FIGURE 2.5
Mean ratings for older adults' preferences for human versus robot assistance (from: Smarr et al., 2014).

adults who were shown a video demonstrating a robot's (Willow Garage's PR2) capabilities and were asked to assume they needed assistance with performing a wide range of tasks (and that the robot could perform the tasks to the level of a human). They rated their preference for assistance for each task on a five-point scale (1 = only a human; 3 = no preference; 5 = only a robot). They had specific preferences for assistance for different tasks. Within each category, the tasks are ordered from greatest mean preference for human assistance to greatest preference for robot assistance. Participants preferred robot assistance rather than human assistance for tasks related to chores, manipulating objects, and information management. They preferred human assistance rather than robot assistance for tasks related to personal care and leisure activities. However, it is important to note that this study only showed them a single robot – preferences likely vary according to the characteristics of the robot, as discussed in Chapter 3. Nevertheless, individual preferences should be considered in the design process.

In our study with professional caregivers, participants were asked to indicate their assistance preference for a robot or human for a wide range of healthcare tasks (on the same scale of 1–5, above; see Figure 2.6). The healthcare tasks were in five categories: activities of daily living, instrumental activities of daily living, nursing activities, medical device use, and communication

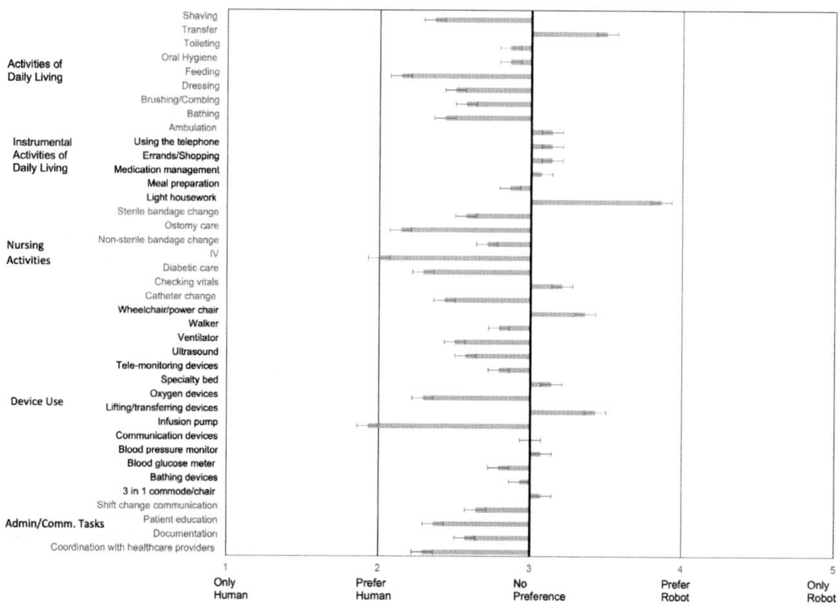

FIGURE 2.6
Mean ratings for professional caregivers' preferences for human versus robot assistance (from: Mitzner et al., 2018).

and administrative activities. Participants were neutral for assistance preference for many of the tasks. However, they preferred a robot assistant for light housework, and they preferred human assistance for IV (intravenous) tasks and infusion pump devices. Such preferences must be considered in the design and deployment of robots to promote acceptance and adoption. If robots are to be used for certain tasks, users may need assurances about safety and reliability.

2.5 Experiences

An individual's prior experience will influence their interaction with a robot. Given that most older adults have not personally interacted with a robot, their attitudes and expectations may be mostly grounded in how they have seen robots portrayed in the media, as discussed in Chapter 1. This edited, polished, and possibly computer-generated imagery may lead to unrealistically high expectations of what a robot can do. In reality, robots can make errors and be just as unreliable as all other technologies.

Older adults have less technology experience, in general, compared to younger adults. Hence, they have less experience to draw from regarding how to interact with advanced technologies such as robots. This lack of experience does not mean that older adults should not be considered as users of robots. In fact, the rate of adoption of technology for older users is growing. Rather, it suggests that older users may need more training and support to have successful interactions with robots. However, this does not mean that future older adults – with more technology experience – will be easily able to interact with robots, because technology advancements will continue. Novel technologies can be challenging to use.

Furthermore, an older adult's prior experience in a domain or performing a task will impact their experience using a robot within that domain and doing that task. For example, imagine an older adult who has a long history of having diabetes and using a blood glucose monitor compared to someone who has recently been diagnosed with diabetes. The person with more experience with the disease and the technology used to track glucose would be more likely to identify an error made by a robot assisting with the task than the person with less experience.

An older adult accumulating more experience using a robot can improve the robot's ability to provide a better experience for their interaction. Over time, a robot could experience and learn about an older adult's demographic background, abilities (strengths as well as challenges), affect, personality, self-efficacy, stress, and preferences. The more complex and rich this understanding is, the more customized interaction the robot could provide.

2.6 Design guidelines for human characteristics

- Given the exponential growth of the aging population, older adults should be considered potential users and included in use cases when developing robots.
- Recognize that demographic characteristics may affect acceptance and use of robots.
- Accommodate age-related perceptual changes.
  - Make sure to use sufficiently sized text and icons, and provide high contrast.
  - Reduce potential for background noise, and avoid high-frequency feedback and alerts.
  - Consider changes in smell, taste, touch, as relevant for the design.
- Consider age-related declines in motor functions (strength, speed, coordination, balance, reaction time, learning).
- Be aware of fall risk – develop robotic applications to decrease fall risk and make sure the robot itself does not impose a risk.
- Remember that older adults hold considerable world knowledge and wisdom.
- Compensate for common age-related cognitive declines, such as memory, by minimizing steps or providing cues about what to do.
- Recognize inter-individual and intra-individual differences in psychosocial characteristics (i.e., affect, personality, self-efficacy, stress, and preferences), as well as age-related changes in emotion regulation.
- Develop robots that can monitor and assess common health conditions, and provide support or intervention for negative affect, poor self-efficacy, stress, and social isolation.
- Provide adequate training and support to facilitate self-efficacy, given that older adults likely have less technology experience.
- Ensure older adults' preferences are addressed in the design of what robots look like and how they provide support.

Recommended readings and links

Readings

Beer, J. M., Prakash, A., Smarr, C.-A., Chen, T. L., Hawkins, K., Nguyen, H., Deyle, T., Mitzner, T. L., Kemp, C. C., & Rogers, W. A. (2017). Older users' acceptance of an assistive robot: Attitudinal changes following brief exposure. *Gerontechnology, 16*, 21–36. https://doi.org/10.4017/gt.2017.16.1.003.00

Boot, W., Charness, N., Czaja, S. J., & Rogers, W. A. (2020). *Designing for older adults: Case studies, methods, and tools*. CRC Press.

Chen, T. L., Bhattacharjee, T., Beer, J. M., Ting, L. H., Hackney, M. E., Rogers, W. A., & Kemp, C. (2017). Older adults' acceptance of a robot for partner dance-based exercise. *PLoS One, 12*(10), e0182736.

Czaja, S. J., Boot, W. R., Charness, N., & Rogers, W. A. (2019). *Designing for older adults: Principles and creative human factors approaches* (3rd ed.). CRC Press.

Czaja, S. J., & Sharit, J. (2012). *Designing training and instructional programs for older adults*. CRC Press.

McLaughlin, A., & Pak, R. (2020). *Designing displays for older adults* (2nd ed.). CRC Press.

Mitzner, T. L., Tiberio, L., Kemp, C. C., & Rogers, W. A. (2018). Understanding healthcare providers' perceptions of a personal assistant robot. *Gerontechnology, 17*, 48–55. https://doi.org/10.4017/gt.2018.17.1.005.00

Prakash, A., & Rogers, W. A. (2015). Why some humanoid faces are perceived more positively than others: Effects of human-likeness and task. *International Journal of Social Robotics, 7*, 309–331.

Smarr, C.-A., Mitzner, T. L., Beer, J. M., Prakash, A., Chen, T. L., Kemp, C. C., & Rogers, W. A. (2014). Domestic robots for older adults: Attitudes, preferences, and potential. *International Journal of Social Robotics, 6*(2), 229–247.

Trifilio, E., Williamson, J. B., & Heilman, K. M. (2020). Changes in emotions and mood with aging. In K. M. Heilman & S. E. Nadeau (Eds.), *Cogn`itive changes and the aging brain* (pp. 127–139). Cambridge University Press.

U.S. Administration for Community Living. (2023). 2023 Profile of Older Americans.

Links

Older Adults Embrace Tech But Are Skeptical of AI (AARP):
https://www.aarp.org/pri/topics/technology/internet-media-devices/2024-technology-trends-older-adults.html

Older Americans 2020: Key indicators of well-being:
https://agingstats.gov/docs/LatestReport/OA20_508_10142020.pdf

Pew Research Center on Older Adults and Technology:
https://www.pewresearch.org/topic/internet-technology/user-demographics/age-generations-tech/older-adults-tech/

Profile of older Americans:
https://acl.gov/aging-and-disability-in-america/data-and-research/profile-older-americans

Putting a face on a robot:
https://phys.org/news/2013-10-robot.html

World Health Organization (WHO) ageing and health:
https://www.who.int/news-room/fact-sheets/detail/ageing-and-health

3

Robot characteristics

3.1 Overview of robot characteristics

Much like humans, robots vary widely in terms of their appearance, capabilities, socialness, and autonomy. As discussed briefly in Chapter 1, robots come in all shapes and sizes, and their technical capabilities have advanced

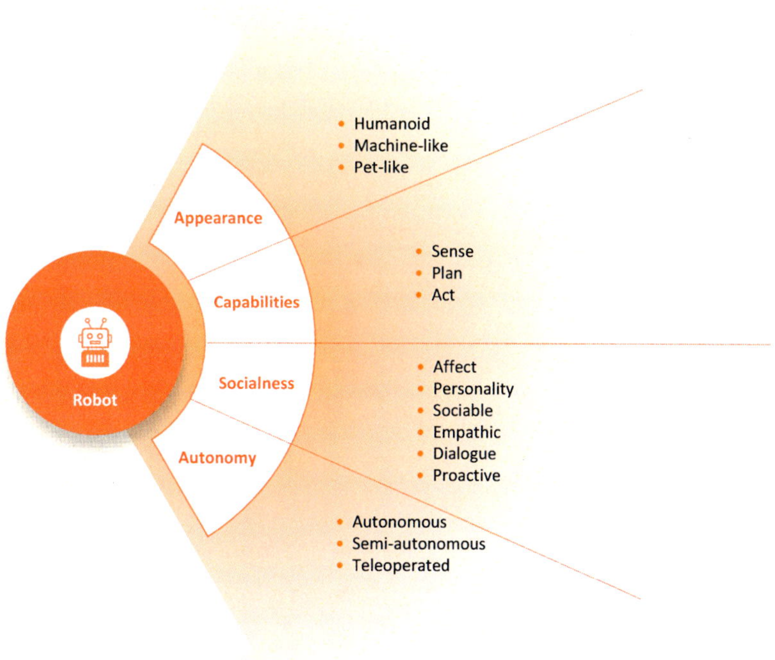

FIGURE 3.1
HRI framework: robot characteristics.

DOI: 10.1201/9781032656649-3

dramatically in the last decade. These characteristics will influence human behavior as well as the successful achievement of the task goals. Figure 3.1 presents this component of our human-robot interaction (HRI) framework.

The robot components in the framework are aspects that should be considered in the design of the robot as well as in the selection of a specific robot for a particular task or person. As when discussing the human, the whole is more than the sum of the parts, and the robot characteristics should be considered holistically in HRI contexts. Nevertheless, it is worthwhile to consider them independently during the design process as well as in research studies to understand the relative impact of different robot characteristics on human behavior and successful task performance.

3.2 Appearance

The most immediately noticeable aspect of the robot is what it looks like. We have defined a robot as being embodied and the physicality will vary widely. The appearance of a robot influences a person's willingness to interact with it initially and continually over time. As well, the appearance will influence enjoyment of the interaction over time, expectations of the robot capabilities, trust, and reliance on the robot. Figure 3.2 presents a collage of robot appearances in three main categories: humanoid, machinelike, and pet-like.

3.2.1 Humanoid

The description *humanoid* is applied to a robot that has some shared characteristics of a human. However, as evident in Figure 3.2, the degree of human-likeness varies widely. Some robots, such as Ameca and Pepper, have a physical form like a human, with arms, legs (or maybe just a base), and a face with expressive capabilities. Others, such as Sophia, are really meant to mimic a human. There is even a trend toward developing robot skins that can mimic the appearance, feel, and sensitivity of human skin.

One challenge encountered in designing humanoid robots is referred to as the "uncanny valley," a term that was coined in 1970 by Masahiro Mori. The uncanny valley theory is a popularized hypothetical relationship of the human-likeness of a robot with the level of familiarity or affinity evoked in the human observer. This relation is posited to be curvilinear: as the appearance of a robot increases in human-likeness, people's familiarity with it increases, but only up to a certain point. Beyond this critical point, a further increase in robot human-likeness results in the robot being perceived as strange or eerie. If the robot's human-likeness can be increased to almost entirely match the appearance of a human, familiarity will presumably rise again and be maximized when the robot cannot be distinguished from a healthy person. The region of dip in familiarity (where the robot is perceived

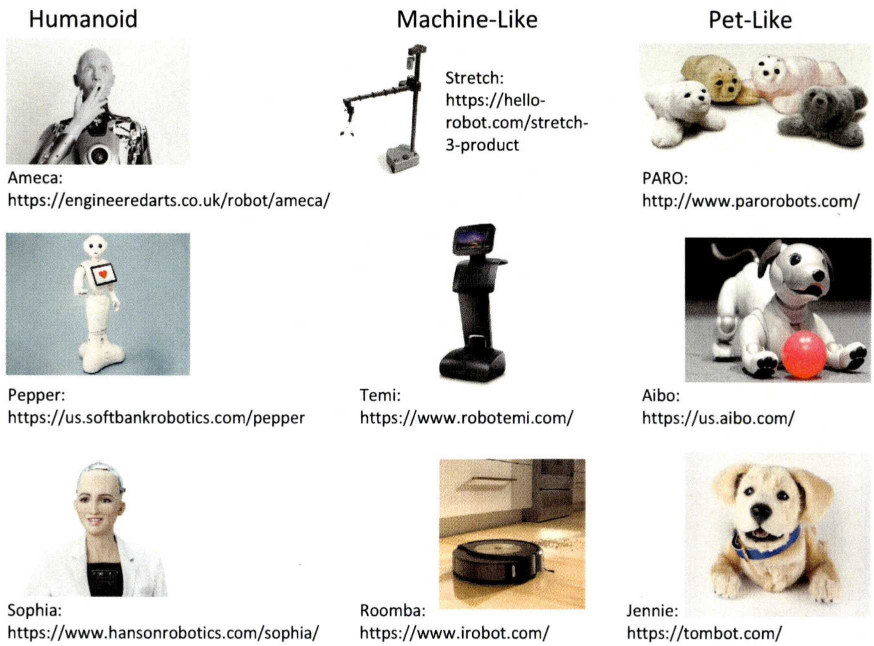

FIGURE 3.2
Robot appearance types.

as strange) with increasing human-likeness is referred to as the uncanny valley (see Figure 3.3).

Although there are mixed views about the generalizability of the uncanny valley phenomenon and limited systematic evidence, there certainly are individual differences in people's preferences for humanlike robots. Interestingly, preferences for appearance interact with the nature of the task that the robot is performing. We found in one study that if the robot was performing chores such as housekeeping, less humanlike robot faces were preferred; on the contrary, for more socially engaging tasks or personal care tasks, more humanlike faces were preferred (Prakash & Rogers, 2015). We will return to the importance of tasks in Chapter 4, but the main point to note here is that not only does appearance affect perceptions, but that preferences vary across tasks as well as across people.

3.2.2 Machinelike

A robot that is *machinelike* is generally made of a hard substance such as Stretch, Temi, and the Roomba depicted in Figure 3.2. Such robots are not intended to look like a human, but they may have some shared characteristics such as the Stretch arm and gripper, which may function like a human arm and hand. Moreover, people may attribute social characteristics to even a machinelike robot without a face. In our work with the Stretch robot, nearly

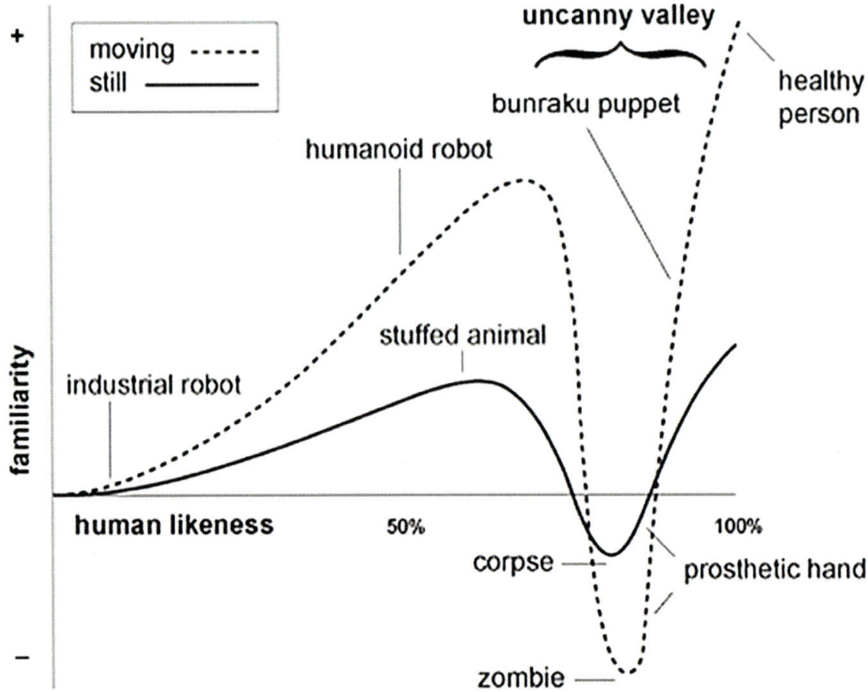

FIGURE 3.3
Hypothesized uncanny valley diagram (from: Mori, 1970; translated by MacDorman & Minato, 2005).

every time Stretch handed a research participant an item, such as a bottle of water, the person would say "thank you." These expectations of interactions may be more likely for human-looking robots but may emerge for a broad range of robots.

Personification and personalization have been observed for machinelike robots. An early example is shown in Figure 3.4. When Roombas were first becoming popular, people started personalizing them with decorations, stickers, logos writing, etc. They reportedly wanted to make it their own. Today, there are after-market items that are specially targeted to Roomba personalization, including custom decals and skins.

3.2.3 Pet-Like

The third general appearance type is *pet-like*, depicted in Figure 3.2 by PARO, Aibo, and Jennie. PARO was designed to mimic a harp seal, perhaps in part to avoid the strong associations people already have with cats and dogs, and hence the risk of the uncanny valley phenomenon. Figure 3.2 also shows two instantiations of robot dogs. The Aibo has the characteristics and personality of a dog but does not physically feel like a dog (i.e., does not have fur). Jennie

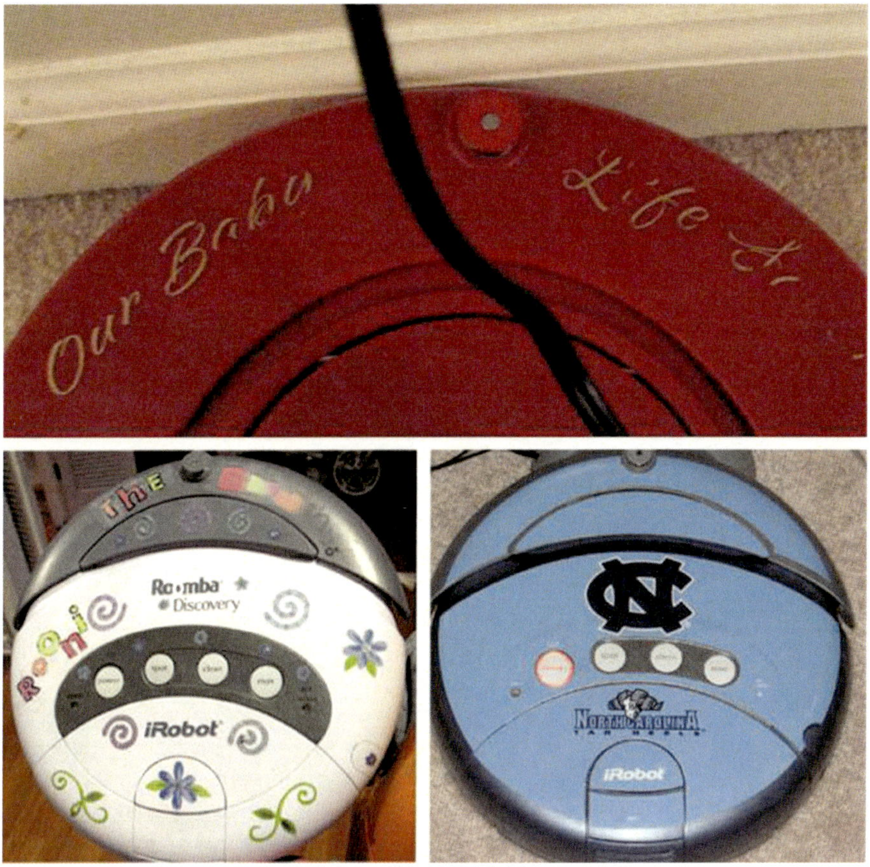

FIGURE 3.4
Illustrations of early Roomba personalization (from: Sung et al., 2009).

is a robot dog, for which great effort has been made to make it feel like a real dog. One thing to keep in mind is the intended purpose of the robot. Both PARO and Jennie are intended to be stroked and held, as one would with a real pet. For other pet-like robots such as Aibo, the intent may be more in the variety of actions that it can do.

3.3 Capabilities

The standard definition of a robot is that it can sense, plan, and act, as we discussed in Chapter 1 (see Figure 1.2). These capabilities are the core of a robot, determining what types of tasks it can perform, the level of precision, the reliability, the fluidity, the complexity, and ultimately the successful achievement of the task goal. Advancements in all areas of engineering (e.g., computer, electrical, mechanical, materials, software, industrial) are contributing to rapid developments of robot capabilities. Our focus here is not on how these capabilities are instantiated from an engineering perspective. Rather the goal is to understand broadly what a robot's capabilities might include.

3.3.1 Sense

A robot can sense aspects of the environment including sights, sounds, smells, textures, temperatures, and motions. In addition, robots can sense stimuli outside of the range of human abilities such as ultraviolet and infrared waves or chemical compositions. A robot can have a wide variety of sensors such as a camera, accelerometer, thermometer, microphone, pressure sensor, gyroscope, chemical detectors, global positioning system, or electromagnetic wave detectors. A given robot might have a small number of sensors, given its functional goals, or multiple sensors in the same category (e.g., various types of cameras located on the robot). Sensors are becoming smaller, faster, more sensitive, and smarter. The technology needed to integrate and coordinate sensor data is developing rapidly.

3.3.2 Plan

What is referred to as the *planning capabilities* of the robot are its abilities to integrate the data from all the sensors into meaningful information that can then guide the robot behaviors. In addition, robots have the capability to store or access vast quantities of information, follow decision-making rules, and carry out complex calculations, usually in real time. For example, motion planning would necessitate awareness of where the robot currently is, the possible directions in which it can move, and the appropriate direction to move given a particular goal (e.g., moving from the kitchen into the bedroom to deliver something to a person). Robots engage in task planning when integrating information and determining the next step in a procedure, or conversation planning when interpreting what a person has said and determining what an appropriate response would be. Robots might have low-level controllers, motion planners, high-level goal planning, learning-based modules, large language models, and much more to support their integration of data and planning processes.

3.3.3 Act

A robot can perform actions in the world, based on what has been sensed and what plan is activated. The actions are numerous, ranging from gross motor movement of the robot through space to fine movements such as the arch of an eyebrow and many things in between. Actuators convert energy into physical motions that enable robots to interact with their environment and perform tasks. The actuators can be electric motors, hydraulic or pneumatic systems, or combinations. Robots can have end effectors, which are peripheral devices that can be attached to a robot's wrist, for example, to allow it to interact in different ways, such as a gripper or a tool.

This summary provides a greatly oversimplified description of what robots can do. Moreover, the sense-act-plan sequence occurs rapidly and is responsive to new information in the environment. From the perspective of the human, these activities may appear seamless, but there is immense processing power supporting the actions of the robot. The human user may not need to know exactly how a robot moves through an environment or what enables it to pick up a particular item. However, for successful HRI, the human will need understand the limitations and capabilities of the robot: what types of spaces can it negotiate, how quickly can it respond, what is the weight limit for an item it can pick up, and what is the basis for the decisions it makes and how reliable are those decisions? In addition, understanding the nature of errors that robots can make, and appropriately calibrating reliance and trust are necessary for humans to interact with robots safely and effectively. Accurate expectations are important for acceptance and adoption.

3.4 Socialness

Socialness is a multifaceted construct in robots, as it is in humans. A robot might engage with a person through voice, text, or pictures; it might display emotions or have a friendly personality; it might be mostly responsive to the human's actions or be proactive in engaging the human in an interaction. In our framework, we have identified the components of socialness that should be considered in the design process and will discuss them in turn. The Moxie robot (https://moxierobot.com/) has many of the social features that a robot might have, and we will use it for illustrating the different components of the framework. On the company website, Moxie is described as follows: "A learning robot with heart, Moxie has endless compassion, unlimited patience, and extensive knowledge." Although Moxie is marketed as being primarily for children, we have found that people of all ages react favorably to the social aspects of it. Figure 3.5 shows a person engaged with Moxie in our home simulation research facility (McKechnie Family LIFE Home; https://lifehome.ahs.illinois.edu/) along with closeups of Moxie's facial expressions. Moxie has voice interaction, which enables it to engage in naturistic dialogue. When we host tours of the LIFE Home, Moxie is always a focal point as visitors become enthralled with the socially interactive experience. To our knowledge, Moxie has not been used in research with older adults, although it has a lot of potential.

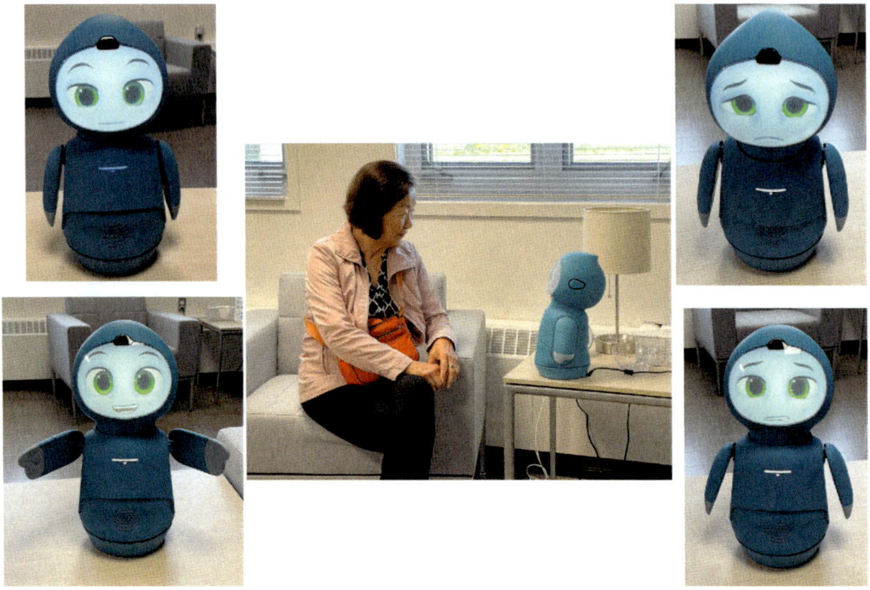

FIGURE 3.5
Person interacting with Moxie (https://moxierobot.com/) and Moxie's facial expressions.

3.4.1 Affect

As we discussed in Chapter 2 in terms of human characteristics, affect can be loosely thought of as feelings, emotions, or mood. As is evident from Figure 3.5, Moxie can display a variety of facial expressions that might be attributed to emotional states such as happy or sad. The idea is for the human to interpret the emotion that the robot is intending to convey. However, given the constraints of the robot embodiment, there may not always be a match between what the design intends to convey and what the person perceives is being displayed.

The Philips iCat was designed to show facial expressions and ultimately be able to develop a relationship between the robot and a human (Van Breemen et al., 2005). We explored the ability of older adults to identify a range of emotions being conveyed by the iCat, as shown in Figure 3.6. Note that in addition to different types of facial expressions, the iCat can show different intensities of emotion; for example, happiness might be displayed as a broad smile, or just a grin. We observed age-related differences in the recognition of emotions expressed by the iCat, with older adults showing lower recognition for the emotions of anger, disgust, fear, happiness, and sadness. These differences might be explained by age-related perceptual changes leading to difficulty discriminating subtle feature differences. For example, older adults often mislabeled fear as surprise. In general, the intensity of the emotion improved recognition.

3.4.2 Personality

A robot can be designed to display a particular personality. For example, Moxie was originally designed for children, and it has an outgoing and playful personality. It is intended to be supportive of the human it interacts with as well as fun to keep them engaged in the interactions. Now consider a robot being used in a healthcare context – this robot may be designed to convey authority, assurance, compassion, kindness, and confidence. Or a robot used in a hotel or restaurant might be outgoing, friendly, and adaptable to a range of people.

The personality characteristics of the robot are often modeled on human characteristics. For instance, what makes a human appear friendly and how can those attributes be instantiated in a robot? Of course, "friendliness" means different things to different people within and across cultures, for different age groups, and perhaps for different levels of cognitive ability. What seems outgoing and fun for one might be perceived as scary or overbearing to another.

3.4.3 Sociable

Sociability is a collective description – it might encompass the affect and personality of a robot as well as its communication style. These components combine to give the robot an overall "sociability" that will influence the human's response to it. Figure 3.7 shows the results of a survey of 51 older adults who watched videos of six different robots (mBot, PR2, Pillo, Relay, Robot.HE, Starship) performing Instrumental Activities of Daily Living (IADL) tasks (i.e., medication management or delivery) with an HRI (i.e., robots were shown interacting with collocated humans). They were asked to provide a rating of their perceptions of the robots' sociability. Then for each robot, they answered questions related to their trust in the robot. As is evident from Figure 3.7, there was a very strong correlation between these two measures (r = .77): the robots

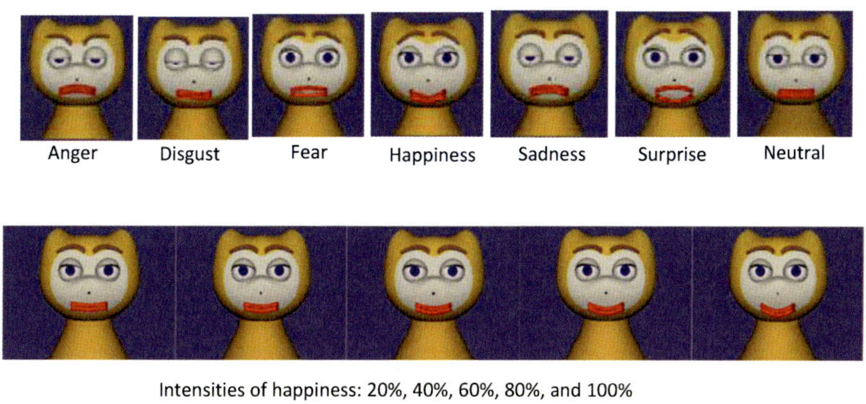

FIGURE 3.6
The iCat robot facial expressions (from: Beer et al., 2015).

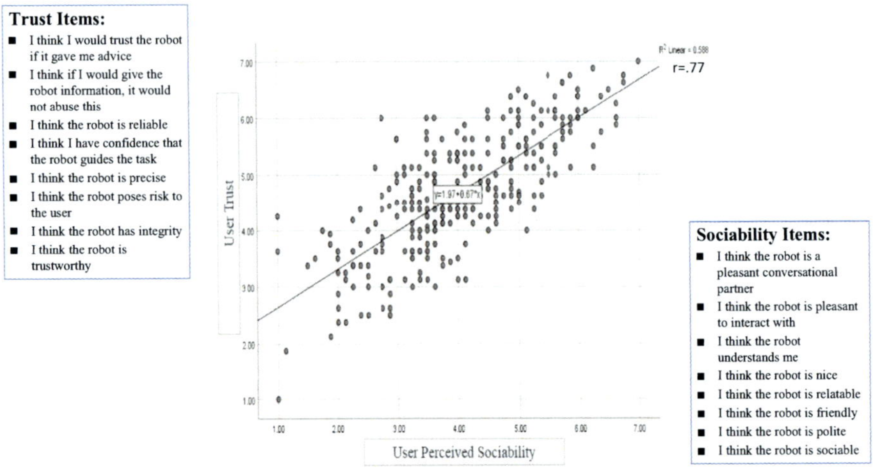

FIGURE 3.7
Participants' ratings of trust in a robot and their perception of sociability of that robot: 1 is strongly disagree, and 7 is strongly agree (from: Kadylak et al., 2023).

perceived as more sociable were trusted more. This finding was replicated in a second sample of 43 older adults that included additional robots (CareoBot, Hollie, PR2, Relay, Stretch), and the correlation between perceived sociability and trust was similarly strong (r = .82).

3.4.4 Empathic

The concept of empathy conveys that the robot is sensitive to the feelings of the person. Empathy can be conveyed by showing an understanding of what the person has said or done and responding appropriately. For example, Moxie might respond to a person saying that they have had a bad day with "I am sorry to hear that you have had a bad day." Or a statement about a joyful experience might be followed by "That's great to hear!" The idea of empathy is that the robot is reacting in a contextually appropriate way to the human. The challenge from the robot side is that it must be able to accurately interpret the human's emotional state, select from appropriate responses, and convey the right level of empathy (i.e., not too understated or overwhelming). Empathy is a complex human behavior that may be challenging to achieve in a robot, especially one that is intended to interact with a range of people.

3.4.5 Dialogue

One aspect of social behavior is the nature of the interaction – how do the robot and the human communicate with each other? With Moxie, there is the sense of a naturalistic conversation, with turn-taking and appropriate responses to spoken statements. However, a human might also be able to type in a command or select from a set of options, and the robot would then respond. This is a type of dialogue between the human and the robot. The nature of the dialogue can vary depending on the capabilities of the robot. For example, it may only have a small set of programmed responses that it can select from, or it may be tapping into large language models in the cloud that make it appear to be socially intelligent.

Digital assistants and artificial intelligence (AI) chatbots (e.g., ChatGPT, watsonx, Copilot) using large language models and natural language processing have advanced the humanlike conversations that robots can have. These generative AI systems enable real-time interactive conversations and can be embedded in robots.

3.4.6 Proactive

An additional component of the socialness of the robot relates to whether it can initiate the interaction. Many robots are dormant until called upon, much like digital assistants that listen for a wake word and then respond (e.g., Alexa, Bixby, Siri). Robots may be similarly programmed to just stand by until called on. For example, Moxie requires the comment "Wake up, Moxie" to initiate the interaction. After that, Moxie can initiate conversations – and in fact will continue to try to engage with the user until it is told "Moxie, go to sleep." The level of proactivity of a robot may be challenging to calibrate to the satisfaction of different users. For example, having a robot start moving and talking to you when you walk in a room may be perceived as comforting and welcoming, or unnerving. As we know from Chapter 2, personalities and preferences differ between humans, which will in turn influence their willingness to interact with different robots.

3.5 Autonomy

The idea that tasks can be allocated between a human and a machine has been actively researched in the field of human factors for many decades. Originally described by Sheridan and Verplank (1978) but often adapted over the years is a list of levels of automation that provides a basis for thinking about human-machine interactions. For example, this list from Sheridan and Parasuraman (2005) can be adapted to show human-robot task allocation.

1. The computer [robot] offers no assistance; the human must do it all.
2. The computer [robot] suggests alternative ways to do the task.
3. The computer [robot] selects one way to do the task and
   - 3a. executes that suggestion if the human approves, or
   - 3b. allows the human a restricted time to veto before automatic execution, or

3c. executes the suggestion automatically, then necessarily informs the human, or

3d. executes the suggestion automatically, then informs the human only if asked.

4. The computer [robot] selects the method, executes the task, and ignores the human.

Moreover, the level of automation and hence robot autonomy can vary from low to high for each robot capability (sense/plan/act) as illustrated in Figure 3.8. And one robot can have different modes of autonomy perhaps for different tasks.

3.5.1 Autonomous

A fully autonomous robot can perform activities without input from a human once the activity is initiated. The robot uses its sensors to perceive the environment, perhaps navigate, make decisions, and perform actions without input from a human. For example, consider the Roomba: once it is programmed to vacuum at a specific time, a person does not have to be available to turn it on, tell it what to do, or turn it off. In this case, the vacuuming can be done when the person is away from home. However, suppose the robot gets stuck under the couch – it will need to be programmed to turn itself off. Or suppose the container for the dirt gets full – the robot may need to send an alert to the user. Autonomy requires advanced levels of safety considerations, error analysis, and built-in fail-safes.

As illustrated in Figure 3.8, aspects of the robot capabilities may be fully autonomous. For example, sensing may be done continuously without need for initiation from a human. Or the planning and selection of options may be completed autonomously. Or an action, once initiated, may be completed autonomously. For example, a robot commanded to go to the bedroom may do so autonomously having learned the layout of the environment, with the ability to avoid obstacles on the way, and awareness of when it has arrived at the desired location.

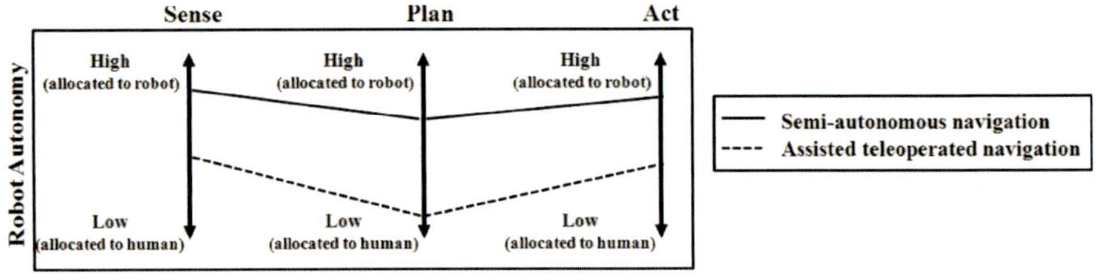

FIGURE 3.8
Levels of robot autonomy (from: Beer et al., 2014).

3.5.2 Semiautonomous

A semiautonomous robot will depend on commands from a human to start, stop, or perform actions in a certain way. For instance, consider a robot delivering an object to a human – it might autonomously identify the person and navigate to where the person is. The human might then instruct the robot about where to put the object (e.g., in their hand or on the table) or indicate when to release the object. This interaction enables the human to rely on the robot for certain aspects of the task (capitalizing on its capabilities) but to control the robot, which may be especially important when the human and the robot must physically interact. A design consideration will be supporting mode awareness for the user (is the robot operating autonomously at the moment) and enabling ease of switching between modes of operation.

3.5.3 Teleoperated

Some robots – or robot actions – may be fully controlled by a human through some type of teleoperation. By definition, teleoperation is to control the robot from a distance. For example, a game controller might be used to move the robot through an environment, actively starting, stopping, turning, or adjusting the robot to exactly where it is intended to be. The control may be of the entire robot, an arm on the robot, or an end effector such as a gripper. Teleoperation may be controlled through an interface using button clicks, mouse dragging/dropping, slider controls, etc. Moreover, teleoperation may occur when the robot is co-located with the robot (i.e., the robot is in sight of the human) or when the human is remotely located and must rely on either cameras or feedback from the robot to calibrate the control.

3.6 Design guidelines for robot characteristics

- Consider the purpose of the robot early in the design process – functionality should be driven by needs and goals.
- Recognize that robot appearance preferences vary across people, contexts, and cultures, and that appearance influences expectations.
- Determine the appropriate type (humanoid, machinelike, pet-like) for your target tasks and users.
- Identify the types of data that will be needed when selecting sensors.
- Evaluate the complexity of use cases for programming the planning capabilities.
- Assess the context of use as well as potential safety concerns when determining the range of robot actions.

- Be aware of the complexity of socialness – consider the affect, personality, empathy, dialog, and proactivity of the robot in terms of the potential users and likely tasks.
- Explore different levels of user control to identify what actions can/should be autonomous, semiautonomous, or teleoperated.
- Recognize that higher levels of human control will require learning and training, whereas higher levels of robot control may require more trust.

Recommended readings and links

Readings

Bayles, M. A., Lee, J., Kadylak, T., & Rogers, W. A. (2023). Understanding older adults' initial perceptions of robot appearance and function: Implications for acceptance. *Gerontechnology, 22*. https://doi.org/10.4017/gt.2023.22.2.bay.08

Beer, J. M., Prakash, A., Smarr, C.-A., Chen, T. L., Hawkins, K., Nguyen, H., Deyle, T., Mitzner, T. L., Kemp, C. C., & Rogers, W. A. (2017). Older users' acceptance of an assistive robot: Attitudinal changes following brief exposure. *Gerontechnology, 16*, 21–36. PMCID: PMC6554728

Goetz, J., Kiesler, S., & Powers, A. (2003). Matching robot appearance and behavior to tasks to improve human-robot cooperation. *The 12th IEEE International Workshop on Robot and Human Interactive Communication Proceedings: ROMAN 2003* (pp. 55–60). https://doi.org/10.1109/ROMAN.2003.1251796

Leng, M, Liu, P., Zhang, P., Hu, M., Zhou, H., Li, G., Yin, H., & Chen, L. (2019). Pet robot intervention for people with dementia: A systematic review and meta-analysis of randomized controlled trials. *Psychiatry Research, 271,* 516–525. https://doi.org/10.1016/j.psychres.2018.12.032

Li, D., Rau, P. L. P. & Li, Y. (2010). A cross-cultural study: Effect of robot appearance and task. *International Journal of Social Robotics,* 2, 175–186. https://doi.org/10.1007/s12369-010-0056-9

Links

Aibo:
https://us.aibo.com/

Ameca:
https://engineeredarts.co.uk/robot/ameca/

Jennie:
https://tombot.com/

McKechnie Family LIFE Home:
https://lifehome.ahs.illinois.edu/

Moxie robot:
https://moxierobot.com/

PARO:
http://www.parorobots.com/

Pepper:
https://us.softbankrobotics.com/pepper

Putting a face on a robot:
https://phys.org/news/2013-10-robot.html

Robot guide:
https://robotsguide.com/robots

Roomba:
https://www.irobot.com/

Sophia:
https://www.hansonrobotics.com/sophia/

Stretch:
https://hello-robot.com/stretch-3-product

Temi:
https://www.robotemi.com/

Types of robots:
https://robotsguide.com/learn/types-of-robots

4

Interaction characteristics

4.1 Overview of interaction characteristics

Any interaction between a robot and an older adult will have unique characteristics depending on the nature of the task, the role the older adult has in the interaction, the engagement characteristics required, and the workload imposed by the task (see Figure 4.1). Interaction characteristics have implications for robot design. For example, a cleaning robot may need to use cleaning tools and products, be supervised by an older user, and apply physical force or load. Alternatively, a bathing robot may need to be operated by an older adult, use products, gently touch the older adult, and work quickly. Moreover, robots can be single-purpose or multipurpose; the more tasks a robot is designed to do, the more complex the set of interaction characteristics that need to be considered. In this chapter, we discuss a range of tasks with which older adults could benefit from having robotic support and provide examples of robots currently available or in development in several categories of tasks. We discuss additional interaction characteristics that may be particularly relevant for robots designed to assist older adults related to roles, engagement, and workload.

4.2 Task

Task characteristics include the type, constraints, device use, and criticality regarding the activity at hand. Many stories in the press highlight the potential of robots to "care for" the rapidly aging society. For example, a 2022 article in *Nature* was titled "Robots rise to meet the challenge of caring for old people" (Savage, 2022). Caregiving is a specific task for which robots show promise, but there is a wide range of tasks beyond caregiving for which robots can support older adults. Moreover, the literature shows clear direction that technological supports for older users should position older adults as active stakeholders in the user experience, rather than only having passive roles and being acted upon by the technology.

DOI: 10.1201/9781032656649-4

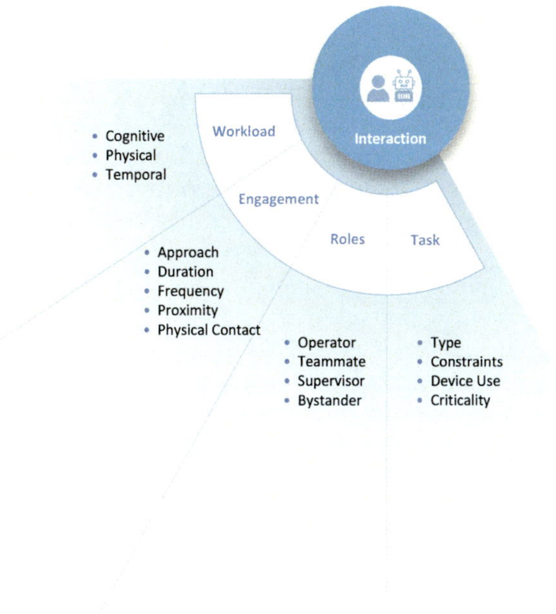

FIGURE 4.1
HRI framework: interaction characteristics.

Robots have much to offer older users in supporting their independence and autonomy. To design useful robots that are likely to be adopted by older users, we must consider the nuances of the activities for which they will need to support. We focus most of this chapter on the different types of tasks that robots have potential to support, those most likely in need of support by older adults, as well as those most important to maintaining independence and a high quality of life. Tasks vary in how critical they are to complete, what constraints are associated, and whether the robot will need to use a device. We provide examples of how these other task characteristics can vary depending on the task type.

4.2.1 Type

One critical predictor of technology adoption is perceived usefulness. To design robots that will be perceived as useful by older adults, we must understand what activities and tasks older adults require support to perform. Older adults prefer to retain their independence no matter where they are living. Regardless of where they live – a long-time home, a senior-living condominium, or an assisted-living apartment – their changing needs and abilities may necessitate support for a range of daily activities. Indeed, needs for support with certain activities are highly correlated with transitions to communities that provide more support, for example, from independent living to assisted living to skilled nursing.

As discussed in Chapter 2, older adults are a diverse population with varying needs, preferences, capabilities, and limitations. Thus, robots designed to support them will likely have to perform a wide range of tasks. We discuss general trends regarding older adults' support needs in different categories of daily living. However, keep in mind the individual characteristics of people, the amount and frequency of support needed, and preferences for how support is provided will vary.

Basic activities of daily living (ADLs) are focused on taking care of one's own body. They include bathing and showering, toileting and toilet hygiene, dressing, eating, functional mobility (including transfer), personal device care, hygiene and grooming, and sexual activity. Given their direct and immediate impact on daily health, these needs must be met for older adults to live independently. Yet, the United States National Health Interview Survey showed that assistance with ADLs is needed for 11% of adults aged 75 or older (see Figure 4.2), and many of these older adults have multiple ADL dependencies.

Typically, the most common needs for support with ADLs include walking, getting in and out of beds and chairs, and bathing and showering. These are mobility-related activities. Mobility support is a crucial need that impacts a large number of older adults. Mobility declines are increasingly prevalent in older adults, with approximately 39% of people aged 65 and older reporting mobility disability (see Figure 2.4), and the risk for disability increasing with

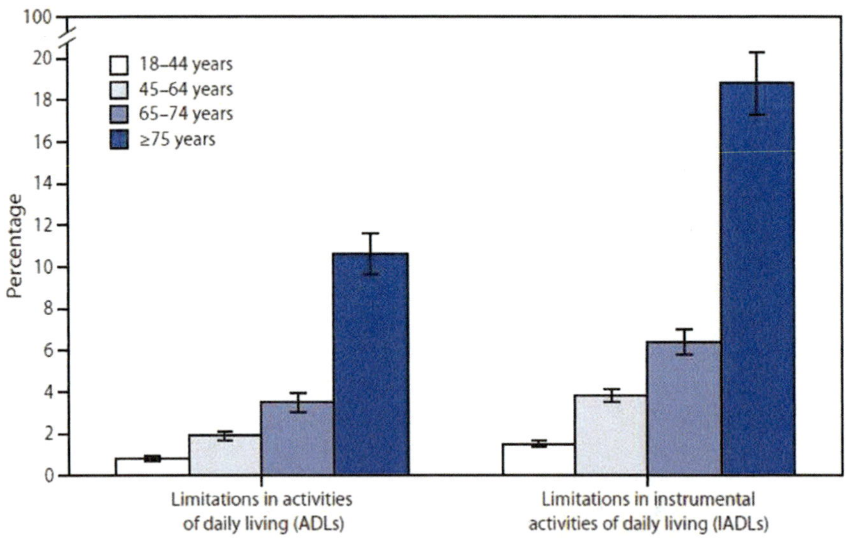

FIGURE 4.2
Limitations in ADLs and IADLs by age (from: National Health Interview Survey, 2014).

age. As a result, the use of mobility aids such as canes, walkers, and wheelchairs (in order of prevalence) is common later in life.

ADLs may require transfers (e.g., bed to chair, chair to toilet), which are associated with risks. Many older adults report difficulty and fear of falls associated with transfer tasks such as toileting. Assistance from another person, such as a care partner or professional caregiver, can improve safety for an older adult, but this assistance often poses risks to the people providing assistance who tend to experience high rates of physical injury. Toileting assistance is one of the most challenging and frequent activities in need of support. Although aids such as lifts, grab bars, and slides are available to facilitate transfer, safety risks remain; even professional caregivers can have safety concerns when using them. Hence, robots that support mobility will not only support independence but could lower mortality risk by reducing falls as well as physical injuries to care partners and professional caregivers.

Most supports developed for ADLs have focused on mobility. Commonly used mobility aids are not technology-based but are classified as durable medical equipment. However, there has been great momentum in developing robotics for mobility support, as described below.

The **Lean Empowering Assistant (LEA)** is a robotic walker developed by Robot Care Systems to provide safety and stability to those with reduced mobility. The force applied on the grips is paired with the motor acceleration. LEA contains sensors that can scan the environment and can navigate autonomously and react intelligently to various conditions. For example, if an object is located on the floor that could be a tripping hazard, the walker will slow down for safety (https://www.clicknl.nl/en/cases-kia-2020-2023/lea/).

Researchers from the Devices for Assisted Living (DALI) project developed a robotic **cognitive walker (cWalker)** that gently guides a person around a building safely. The device takes corrective actions when the user comes across potential safety hazards such as a busy area, obstacle, or incident. The c-Walker is equipped with brakes and motorized wheels and uses a range of technologies (e.g., Radio Frequency Identification (RFID) tags, invisible Quick Response (QR) codes, cameras) to localize itself in the environment. It can also connect with remote sensors such as surveillance cameras to gain remote knowledge of the presence of crowded spaces or hazards. Haptic armbands tell users when and how to turn and can call for assistance if needed (http://www.ict-dali.eu/news.html).

Developers from Nanyang Technological University (NTU) in Singapore, developed a **Mobile Robotic Balance Assistant (MRBA)**. It looks like a motorized wheelchair with guard rails that come up to a person's hip and is embedded with sensors to determine when a person begins to lose their balance. Users strap into a harness, and when they are starting to lose their balance, the robot engages to keep them from falling (https://www.ntu.edu.sg/mae/news-events/news/detail/mae-prof-invents-mobile-robotic-balance-assistant).

Lifeward has developed two robotic mobility aids. **ReWalk** is a wearable robotic exoskeleton that provides powered hip and knee motion to enable individuals with spinal cord injury to stand upright, walk, turn, and climb/descend stairs. ReWalk is the first exoskeleton to receive Food and Drug Administration (FDA) clearance in the United States for personal and rehabilitation use. **ReStore** is a powered, lightweight, soft exo-suit designed for rehabilitation purposes for individuals with lower limb disability due to stroke. It is the only post-stroke gait training tool that provides both dorsiflexion (flexing your foot so that your toes move toward your body) and plantarflexion (movement of pointing your toes away from your body) assistance to facilitate functional gait training (https://golifeward.com/products/).

The **Robot for Interactive Body Assistance (RIBA)** was developed by RIKEN-SRK Collaboration Center for Human-Interactive Robot Research and Sumitomo Riko Company in Japan to assist transfer by lifting people out of their beds and wheelchairs and transferring them to new positions. RIBA was designed to look friendly and "hug" patients in the transferring process. Although it still requires a caregiver to provide navigational assistance, it has the potential to reduce falls for the older adults and musculoskeletal injuries for the caregiver or care partner (http://rtc.nagoya.riken.jp/RIBA/index-e.html).

The **Autobed** is a repositioning bed designed by Georgia Tech researchers. It provides an accessible web-based control to reposition an electric bed. The design instructions are open-source, so that anyone can develop their own autobed with a hospital bed and a web interface (https://sites.gatech.edu/hrl/autobed-a-web-controlled-robotic-bed/).

Panasonic has demonstrated a **robotic hair washing device** that applies shampoo and hot water, and gently massages the scalp (https://news.panasonic.com/global/press/en110926-2).

Obi was developed to provide feeding assistance. It has five depths of fields to scoop food up and bring it to the user's mouth after training (https://meetobi.com/).

A **meal-assistance system** was developed by Georgia Tech researchers to use with a general-purpose mobile manipulator (the Willow Garage PR2). The active feeding system enables the robot to autonomously deliver food to a user's mouth, minimizing the need for head movement by the user. The system incorporates a user interface, visually guided behavior, and safety tools to allow people with even severe motor impairments to successfully use the system.

Robots that can assist with wide-ranging ADL tasks could have life-changing impacts on quality of life. Robots could enable an individual with quadriplegia to feed themselves or move their body position, supporting their own autonomy and providing respite for a care partner. Or for an individual who needs support with only one ADL (e.g., toileting), robots could enable the person to delay needing a professional caregiver or moving to assisted living.

Instrumental activities of daily living (IADLs) include caring for others and pets, communication management, driving and community mobility, financial management, health management and maintenance, home establishment and management, meal preparation and cleaning, religious and spiritual activities and expressions, safety procedure and emergency responses, and shopping. Almost 20% of persons aged 75 or older require assistance for

IADLs (see Figure 4.2), most commonly for housekeeping and maintenance tasks, meal preparation, and health/medication management.

Housekeeping tasks include washing dishes, doing laundry, changing linens, emptying trash cans, taking trash and recycling bins to the curb, dusting, cleaning windows, as well as vacuuming, sweeping, and mopping floors. Maintenance tasks include ensuring home security, testing alarms and detectors, replacing air filters, cleaning vent ducts, cleaning window screens, and painting. Our research has shown that older adults report difficulties with many of these tasks including cleaning gutters, painting the exterior of their home, cleaning floors, and changing bed linens (see Figure 4.3). Cleaning and maintenance tasks are often physically demanding and may involve having to reach high and low places in the home. Activities such as gutter cleaning, window washing, and painting are associated with safety risks such as falls from ladders. Falls from ladders can cause severe injuries, particularly for older adults. The physical demands of home cleaning and maintenance tasks can reduce the time and energy an individual has available for more enjoyable activities.

Health management and maintenance tasks include managing acute and chronic conditions, facilitating rehabilitation from injury, and managing healthcare provider appointments, medications, and wellness activities. Older adults' health needs might include support for acute illnesses as well as for chronic conditions. Almost all adults aged 60 and older have at least one chronic condition, and many have two or more. The most common conditions associated with those aged 65 and over are hypertension, high cholesterol, arthritis, heart disease, diabetes, chronic kidney disease, heart failure, depression, Alzheimer's disease and dementia, and chronic pulmonary disease (see Figure 2.3).

Medication is used to treat many chronic conditions; however, there are challenges to medication adherence including remembering to take medication and then remembering if it has been taken. An additional complication

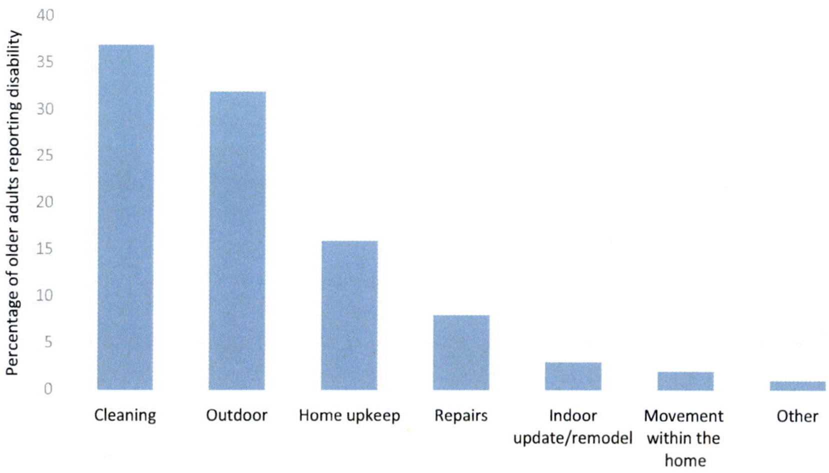

FIGURE 4.3
Maintenance tasks reported as difficult by older adults (adapted from: Fausset et al., 2011).

is that many older adults take multiple mediations. One study found that 39% of adults over 65 take five or more daily medications (Kantor et al., 2015). Not surprisingly, estimated prevalence of medication nonadherence is over 30% in older adults (Liu et al., 2023). Stroke, falls, and injuries increase in prevalence with age, often necessitating rehabilitation services. Lastly, wellness activities, such as engaging in exercise, eating nutritious foods, and managing stress, are important for older adults to engage in to prevent and manage chronic conditions.

Assistance with household tasks has been an attractive use case for robotic assistance predicted as early as the *Jetsons* television show in the early 1960s. This is an application for which we have seen substantial growth, not only in the development of such "domestic" robots but also in their accessibility (e.g., commercial availability, cost). In a recent forecasting study, 65 artificial intelligence (AI) experts from the United Kingdom and Japan were asked to estimate the extent to which various housework tasks would be automated in the future. They estimated that 39% of the time spent performing a household/domestic task would be able to be automated by 2033 (Lehdonvirta et al., 2023). Most commercially available (and adopted) robots developed for supporting IADLs have focused on housekeeping tasks.

In 2002, iRobot released the first commercially successful robotic vacuum cleaner, the **Roomba** (see Figure 3.2). Since then, iRobot has sold more than 40 million robots worldwide. The Roomba is an AI-powered robot vacuum that detects and avoids common robot obstacles, such as cords and cables. iRobot has also developed robotic mops and combination vacuum/mops. Currently, there are many commercially available robotic vacuums and mops available including those sold by Roborock, Eufy, and Shark.

Robotic window cleaners are available such as the **Ecovac Winbot**. These robots use powerful suction systems to allow them to cling to vertical surfaces. Advanced algorithms and intelligent navigation systems guide them, and motorized brushes and cleaning pads work together in the cleaning process (https://www.ecovacs.com/us/winbot-window-cleaning-robot).

Pria, launched by Black+Decker, is an automated medication management and home healthcare assistant device. It is a voice-enabled tabletop robot that provides caregivers and care partners information about an older adult's daily medication adherence to both prescribed and over-the-counter medications. The system can schedule up to 28 doses and provides reminder alerts, dispenses medication at the scheduled time, and provides the user with quick access to family or caregivers using voice commands and video calls (https://www.okpria.com/).

Wyss startup **Imago Rehab** developed a soft robotic glove for at-home rehabilitation for stroke survivors. The glove provides stretching and repetitive exercises required to restore lost hand function. It has a minimalist form factor so users can keep it on during daily activities. Sensors in the glove collect feedback that can be sent to an occupational therapist, who can monitor and modify the rehabilitation program (https://wyss.harvard.edu/technology/soft-robotic-glove/).

Pepper is a robot personal trainer that can be used to coach runners through an exercise program on a treadmill (see Figure 3.2). Pepper can tell jokes and express sympathy. It provides personalized instruction and feedback based on the user's heart rate, speed, personality type, mood, and fitness level. Pepper was trained by a human fitness instructor on how to be an encouraging coach, learning when to offer praise during a workout and what cues can motivate a person to improve performance (https://us.softbankrobotics.com/pepper).

Robots designed to assist with IADL tasks can greatly impact an individual's independence and well-being. Imagine an older adult whose main challenge is managing their medications. Their nonadherence could lead to unnecessary hospital admissions or even death. Robot support for this task would enable them to age in place and reduce the financial burden associated with additional hospital visits. Robotic support for home cleaning/maintenance and meal preparation could improve an older adult's safety as well as increase the time and energy they have to engage in other more enjoyable and meaningful activities.

Enhanced activities of daily living (EADLs) go beyond maintaining independence in older adulthood and contribute to one's well-being and quality of life. They are activities that are required to maintain an active lifestyle and may include leisure (e.g., watching television, performing hobbies, traveling), social (e.g., social or religious groups or events, playing games with friends and family), physical (e.g., gardening, dancing, golf), and cultural (going to museums, theaters, symphony) activities as well as use of technology (e.g., social media, online shopping) and intellectual pursuits. Given they are more complex activities, EADLs can be difficult to engage in or frustrating because of age-related declines in motor, vision, hearing, or cognition or due to limited technical knowledge.

This category of daily activities is the largest and most individualized across people. An underlying theme of many EADLs is that they have a social component, and socially engaging activities are important to health. Recently, the impact of social isolation on health has become more understood, including increasing negative health outcomes and mortality risk. Unfortunately, feeling isolated in older age is not uncommon. Barriers to social interaction include poor physical health, low education level, low socioeconomic status, low self-esteem, depression, and low technology competence and self-efficacy. Given these findings, older adults have a crucial need for support in social engagement. The context of an individual's needs for support for social engagement can vary greatly and may include both peers and family (i.e., intergenerational) and may take place at home or in the community (i.e., community participation).

Other EADLs that older adults may need assistance with include work, volunteering, and caregiving. Work trends are changing, with more people delaying retirement or going back into the workforce. Older adulthood can be a time of more volunteering, which can improve physical and mental health (e.g., stress reduction) and reduce depression and anxiety. Needs for support for work and volunteering tasks may include assistance with using technology, project management, or completing hazardous or physically challenging tasks.

Many older adults provide caregiving to a spouse or family member. Caregiving tasks range from providing assistance with daily activities and direct care to navigating complex health care and social service systems. Tasks such as transfer, dressing, and bathing are physically demanding and can increase risk for falls or injuries. Even less physical tasks can place demands that increase risk for psychological distress (e.g., anxiety or depressive symptoms) and adverse health outcomes for care partners.

Nevertheless, these negative outcomes can be minimized with provision of needed supports. Intervention studies have shown improvement in care partner health and well-being when their needs are addressed. Tasks that robots could support include provision of knowledge and information about the target disease and available support services, as well as social support, formal therapeutic strategies, and care recipient monitoring.

Robotic supports for EADLs include those designed to provide social interaction and support, as well as physical (e.g., dancing) and mobility support. We provide a sampling here.

ElliQ is a robot that provides conversation about a variety of topics (e.g., news, inspirational quotes, weather, interesting facts, sports updates, music, holiday celebrations, jokes, games) and connection to family and friends (e.g., video calls, connected picture frame, memory sharing, digital greeting cards). It also provides health and wellness supports. States including Florida, Michigan, and Washington are deploying ElliQ robots in an effort to address loneliness in their older residents. New York conducted a two-year pilot project deploying approximate 900 ElliQ robots to older residents. They reportedly found a 95% reduction in loneliness as well as high levels of engagement over time and have now adopted the program statewide (New York State Office for the Aging, 2023; https://elliq.com/).

Telepresence robots, such as the **Double 3** and **Beam**, can facilitate visits to museums or other cultural locations. They can be used to visit a friend or family member who is in another location. Telepresence robots can be operated from a phone, tablet, or computer browser from home, allowing someone to independently navigate a remote space. Case studies of this application include the Massachusetts Museum of Contemporary Art, Hastings Contemporary Art Museum, and Anchorage Museum (https://www.doublerobotics.com/ and https://suitabletech.com/home).

PARO is a robotic companion animal designed to resemble a baby harp seal (including their sounds; see Figure 3.2). It is embedded with five kinds of sensors: tactile, light, audition, temperature, and posture sensors, with which it can perceive people and its environment. PARO can recognize being stroked or held as well as the direction of voice and words (e.g., greetings, praise). It has been shown to have multiple therapeutic effects including stress reduction (http://www.parorobots.com/).

Jennie, developed by Tombot, is a robotic pet dog designed to help people cope with health adversities including stress, anxiety, loneliness, and depression (see Figure 3.2). The dog is embedded with touch sensors to allow her to react based on how and where she is being touched. She has voice activation software that enables her to react to commands. Jennie has realistic sounds that are based on recordings from a 12-week-old Labrador puppy (https://tombot.com/blogs/investors/meet-jennie).

EADLs are an exciting area for future robot support. Robots designed to assist with EADLs can provide opportunities for physical, emotional, and cognitive growth, and improve quality of life and feelings of fulfillment. There is growing research documenting the benefits of robots for supporting the social and cognitive health of older adults. However, there is certainly potential that needs to be investigated further given that robots can provide social (e.g., companionship, facilitating communication with friends and family) and cognitive (e.g., providing puzzles, quizzes, and other cognitively engaging games) stimulation while supporting EADL tasks.

4.2.2 Constraints

Constraints may be imposed by the details of a task, such as whether it is a dynamic task with multiple changing parameters. For example, a telepresence robot that a human is navigating through a complex environment might contain objects as well as other people or pets. This scenario could be for an ADL task such as assisting with ambulation, for an IADL task such as getting someone's medications from a dispenser, or for an EADL task such as playing hide-and-seek with a grandchild remotely. The social context can impose constraints such as etiquette expectations and social norms about performing a behavior. Constraints can be imposed by the robot, including operating conditions, navigational boundaries, and surface requirements. A heavy robot without stairclimbing ability will not be able to assist someone above the ground floor. A robot without fine motor skills and small grippers would not be able to assist someone with putting on a necklace with a small clasp. The environment can impose constraints such as limited space for a robot to move around. Lastly, the older adult can elicit constraints such as the speed at which a robot guides them if they have mobility limitations.

4.2.3 Device use

For some tasks, a robot may need to use a device, such as an appliance, tablet, wearable device, or medical equipment. For example, an individual who does not have the use of their arms may need a robot to use a spoon to feed them to assist with this ADL task. The prevalence of both diabetes and hypertension increases with age (see Figure 2.3). A robot that is providing assistance for managing these chronic conditions, which is an IADL task, may need to use a blood glucose meter or blood pressure monitor. Alternatively, a robot assisting with a hobby such as gardening, an EADL task, may need to use a garden hoe or shovel. The ability to use these devices is going to require that the robot have certain levels of dexterity and maneuverability.

4.2.4 Criticality

Tasks can have different levels of criticality, speed, or accuracy requirements. The degree to which performing a task correctly or not may have serious consequences to one's life or well-being. The criticality of a task will impose constraints on robotic support. Whether a robot folds a towel a certain way would have low criticality. However, the consequence of an error with ADL tasks (e.g., bathing, mobility, transfer) could be very serious for older adults, such as an injurious fall. This type of assistance must be as error-proof as possible and have appropriate safety measures.

Robotic assistance with IADLs such as medication management or financial management has critical consequences for errors. Medication nonadherence accounts for large numbers of hospital admissions and nursing home admissions.

A robotic assistant for an EADL hobby such as woodworking could have critical consequences for errors in the event it is helping someone use a table saw or other dangerous tools. The need for assurances and high thresholds of reliability will be greater for tasks with high criticality than for less critical tasks.

4.3 Roles

The roles that an older adult takes in an HRI experience include being an *operator, teammate, supervisor,* and/or *bystander.* Their role may be dictated by various factors including the task, the user's technology and robot experience, or the user's cognitive status. As an *operator* of a robot, an older adult may be involved in the setup of the robot, performance of tasks using the robot, and maintenance of the robot. This role would be one of the most demanding in terms of knowledge and technology experience and would therefore require more training for the older adult user. This scenario would be similar to the role of an operator of a computer or smartphone. After purchasing the robot, the older adult would need to follow the instructions to set it up and use it and would need to problem solve any technical issues that arise. Hence, the requisite training would need to include the setup and maintenance tasks in addition to the use of the robot to perform tasks and troubleshooting. As with computers and smartphones, some older adults would need assistance at times from a professional, family member, or friend.

Operating a robot may include providing demonstration and feedback to the robot or to customize or refine an action or movement, which can be done using a method called Learning from Demonstration (LfD) or Robot Programming by Demonstration (PbD). The older adult would show the robot how they would like the task to be performed, and the robot would be "programmed" by watching. For example, an older adult could demonstrate how they like their clothes folded so the robot could perform the task that same way in the future. There is growing interest in this method for programming and operating robots as a result of rapid innovation in generative AI, which could dramatically increase the rate at which robots could learn from demonstration.

Alternatively, an older adult may be acting as a *teammate* with the robot, in which case they would share the same goal but may perform different tasks to achieve that goal. That is, they may act as a collaborator or cooperator with the robot. As a collaborator, they would share the same sub-goals and overall goal and have the same hierarchical level as the older adult. The teammate-as-collaborator role might require greater training, particularly if an older adult and robot are performing an action together in real time. The human would need to know how to coordinate with the robot's part of the task. An example would be someone folding a large blanket with a robot. As a cooperator, the human and robot would have different sub-goals but the same overall goals, and the task would be strictly allocated between the human and the robot. An example would be a robot and an older adult cleaning the kitchen together, with the older adult cleaning the easy-to-reach surfaces and the robot cleaning hard-to-reach high and low surfaces. As discussed in Chapter 3, in this example the robot may be acting semi-autonomously, enabling the human to rely on the robot for only certain aspects of the task while maintaining personal autonomy for other aspects of the task. This approach would capitalize on the robot's capabilities (and compensate for the person's limitations) to complete a task together as teammates. Although the word "teammate" is used in the literature, note that use of such anthropomorphic language could trigger unrealistic expectations particularly for an older adult with limited technology and robot experience.

An older adult may act primarily as the *supervisor* of a robot, such as a floor cleaning robot that a residential living community uses to clean its residents' rooms. In this case, less training would be required, but the user would still need to know how to ensure safety and perhaps provide feedback on task performance.

Lastly, an older adult might act simply as a *bystander*, while robots perform a task, in which case training may not be needed but safety considerations would still need to be addressed. For example, a medication robot could be delivering medication to someone and pass by that person's spouse. With both the supervisor and bystander roles, the human would need to know how to stay out of the robot's way.

4.4 Engagement

An older adult's interaction with a robot will be impacted by aspects of their physical engagement such as the *approach* of the robot, the *duration* and *frequency* of interaction, the *proximity* of the robot with respect to the user, and whether *physical contact* is involved. The *approach* of the robot can be impacted by the type of surface it is operating on and whether obstacles or hazards are present. For example, if a robot is assisting with transfer from a seated position to a walker, it may need to approach from the rear or side of the user.

The *duration* of engagement between an older adult and a robot would depend on how much physical interaction is required for the task or how much feedback is required. For a task that involves physical interaction such as bathing, the duration of engagement might be relatively short. However, for a social support task, the duration of engagement could extend for several hours or an entire day.

The *frequency* of the engagement could be low, such as monthly (e.g., testing smoke detectors) or yearly (e.g., securing steps and handrails) home maintenance tasks, or high, such as trip hazard detection and fall monitoring.

The *proximity* between an older adult and robot may vary by task. The robot and the human may be operating in the same physical space or in different spaces (e.g., an older adult controlling a telepresence robot in a remote space), and the robot may need to get within a foot or maybe even a few inches for certain tasks (e.g., to hand off a medication).

For many ADL tasks, *physical contact* is required. The older adult may have to physically touch the robot and vice versa. The need for physical contact will guide the need for sensors on the robot, as well as the structure of the robot (e.g., skin that is reactive to touch, soft grippers so as not to scratch a person). A shower/bathing assistant robot may be more accepted (and safe) if it has soft tactile features, whereas a lawn mowing robot might be more accepted if it looks strong and durable. If the robot is lifting or supporting the person, then factors such as payload, stability, and maneuverability will be relevant.

4.5 Workload

Cognitive workload refers to the amount of thinking, deciding, or calculating necessary for a human to interact with a robot. An overload can lead to diminished performance, errors, and mistakes. Cognitive workload can be impacted by a variety of factors, including the cognitive capacity of the user, whether the user is engaged in more than one task at a time, and the environmental characteristics (e.g., whether stress or distractions are present). Consider a high-stress scenario in the context of an interaction between a robot and an older user (e.g., an older adult has just been notified that their blood pressure is dangerously high). Given that high stress can be cognitively demanding, there would be fewer cognitive resources available to interact with the robot. Poor usability can overload cognitive workload. Usability should be a high priority for older adults because they have less technology experience. However, robots are often designed by younger adults without input from older users.

Physical workload includes the physical demands or intensity of the physical interaction with the robot. An overly demanding physical workload can cause fatigue, diminished task performance, or injury. Robots range in size and weight, sometimes as a design necessity. A window-washing robot must be light enough for a user to move it from window to window (unless it can move itself). A robot that must lift heavy objects or a person must weigh enough to carry that heavy payload. One scenario that must be considered for a robot providing assistance to an older adult is that it may need to be stable enough (and weigh enough) to support the user if they begin to fall and reach out to it for support. If the person lives in a home with stairs and the robot needs to move or be moved from floor to floor, it must be lightweight or be able to move between floors by itself. Alternatively, there could be different robots for each floor.

Temporal workload refers to time-related aspects (e.g., time pressure) that are required to successfully interact with a robot. These demands involve factors such as deadlines, time constraints, scheduling, and prioritization. The temporal workload can relate to other interaction characteristics such as criticality. Some high criticality tasks are also time-sensitive, such as a robot detecting that an older adult has had a stroke or injurious fall. Medication management is time- and schedule-sensitive and a high priority task given the risks and prevalence of nonadherence. Assistance with planning appointments and social events also needs to adhere to time constraints and scheduling issues.

4.6 Design guidelines for interaction characteristics

- Always treat the older adult as an active stakeholder and user.
- Assess and clearly define what tasks need to be supported and what aspects of the task should be supported to maximize older adults' autonomy.
- Consider robot applications to support all types of activity categories (ADL, IADL, EADL).
- Evaluate task constraints such as the physical environment (e.g., stairs, clutter, room size) and the social environment (e.g., pets, care partners, friend and family visitors, social norms). See Chapter 5 for more details about interaction environments.
- Ensure the robot can use devices if needed for the task (e.g., medical devices, home maintenance tools, cooking utensils).
- Pay particular attention to safety for high criticality tasks (medication management, mobility/transfer tasks), adding extra layers of safety if possible (e.g., multiple checks, backup systems).
- Determine the appropriate user's role based on task requirements and the user's capabilities and experience.
- Evaluate needs as well as preferences for engagement characteristics such as the approach, duration, frequency, and proximity of the physical engagement.
- Ensure any physical contact is safe and acceptable.
- Engage older users early and often in the design process to determine cognitive, physical, and temporal workload.

Recommended readings and links

Readings

Ajaykumar, G., & Huang, C. M. (2023). Older adults' task preferences for robot assistance in the home. arXiv preprint. https://arxiv.org/abs/2302.12686

Ajaykumar, G., Pineda, K. T., & Huang, C. M. (2023). Older adults' expectations, experiences, and preferences in programming physical robot assistance. *International Journal of Human-Computer Studies, 180*, 103127.

Beer, J. M., Prakash, A., Smarr, C. A., Mitzner, T. L., Kemp, C. C., & Rogers, W. A. (2012a, September). "Commanding your robot" older adults' preferences for methods of robot control. *Proceedings of the Human Factors and Ergonomics Society Annual Meeting, 56*(1), 1263–1267.

Beer, J. M., Smarr, C. A., Chen, T. L., Mitzner, T. L., Kemp, C. C., & Rogers, W. A. (2012b). The domesticated robot: Design guidelines for assisting older adults to age in place. *Proceedings of the 7th IEEE/ACM International Conference on Human-Robot Interaction* (HRI'12), Boston, MA, pp. 335–342. https://doi.org/10.1145/2157689.2157806

Nolan, E. (2024). For older people who are lonely, is the solution a robot friend? *The New York Times*. https://www.nytimes.com/2024/07/06/nyregion/ai-robot-elliq-loneliness.html

Rogers, W. A., Mitzner, T. L., & Bixter, M. T. (2020). Understanding the potential of technology to support enhanced activities of daily living (EADLs). *Gerontechnology, 19*(2), 125–137.

Smarr, C. A., Mitzner, T. L., Beer, J. M., Prakash, A., Chen, T. L., Kemp, C. C., & Rogers, W. A. (2014). Domestic robots for older adults: Attitudes, preferences, and potential. *International Journal of Social Robotics, 6*, 229–247.

Wolff, J. L., Feder, J., & Schulz, R. (2016). Supporting family caregivers of older Americans. *The New England Journal of Medicine, 375*(26), 2513–2515. https://doi.org/10.1056/NEJMp1612351

Wolinsky, F. D., Bentler, S. E., Hockenberry, J., Jones, M. P., Obrizan, M., Weigel, P. A. M., Kaskie, B., & Wallace, R. B. (2011). Long-term declines in ADLs, IADLs, and mobility among older Medicare beneficiaries. *BMC Geriatrics, 11*, 43.

Links

Autobed:
https://sites.gatech.edu/hrl/autobed-a-web-controlled-robotic-bed/

Beam telepresence:
https://suitabletech.com/home

Cognitive Walker (cWalker) mobility assistant:
http://www.ict-dali.eu/news.html

Double 3 telepresence:
https://www.doublerobotics.com/

Ecovac Winbot window cleaner:
https://www.ecovacs.com/us/winbot-window-cleaning-robot

ElliQ care companion:
https://elliq.com/

Imago Rehab:
https://wyss.harvard.edu/technology/soft-robotic-glove/

Jennie companion animal:
https://tombot.com/blogs/investors/meet-jennie

LEA (Lean Empowering Assistant) mobility assistant:
https://www.clicknl.nl/en/cases-kia-2020-2023/lea/

Mobile Robotic Balance Assistant (MRBA):
https://www.ntu.edu.sg/mae/news-events/news/detail/mae-prof-invents-mobile-robotic-balance-assistant

Obi:
https://meetobi.com/

PARO companion animal:
http://www.parorobots.com/

Pepper personal trainer:
https://us.softbankrobotics.com/pepper

Pria medication manager:
https://www.okpria.com/

ReStore Exo-Suit:
https://golifeward.com/products/restore-exo-suit/

ReWalk Personal Exoskeleton:
https://golifeward.com/products/rewalkpersonal-exoskeleton/

Robot for Interactive Body Assistance (RIBA):
https://www.riken.jp/en/news_pubs/research_news/pr/2009/20090827/

Robotic hair washing device:
https://news.panasonic.com/global/press/en110926-2

Roomba vacuums:
https://www.irobot.com

Soft robotic glove:
https://wyss.harvard.edu/technology/soft-robotic-glove/

5

Interaction environments

5.1 Overview of interaction environments

The context of human–robot interaction (HRI) will impact the interaction, including the environmental context (i.e., natural, built, social, and technology environments; see Figure 5.1). Robots designed for older users may need to traverse or interact with the natural environment (e.g., walking outside, gardening). They may be located in private homes (e.g., single-family and multifamily), communal living settings (e.g., independent living, long-term care residences), clinics, and hospitals. The social environment will vary as a result. Robots will need to be integrated with everyday technologies as they are becoming ubiquitous, including smart home and transportation technologies. In this chapter, we discuss characteristics of different natural, built, social, and technology environments that are likely to be relevant for older adults. Later, in Chapter 8, we describe interaction environments in the context of a private home for a specific case study.

5.2 Natural

The natural environment refers to all non-human-made surroundings, living and nonliving, including the earth, air, water, plants, and animals. We might not immediately think about the relevance of a robot's interaction with the natural environment. If we imagine a robot in a physical space, it is more likely to be that of a building or home, but even indoors natural elements do exist. The robot may be watering indoor plants or taking care of an indoor pet. It could clean a cat's litter box, which can be difficult for older adults as it requires bending and possibly lifting; it could clean the paws of dog coming in from outdoors, which also involves bending, or it could clean a fish tank, which can be physically difficult. Even if robots will not be directly caring for a pet, they need to be pet-friendly and not pose safety issues for pet companions.

 DOI: 10.1201/9781032656649-5

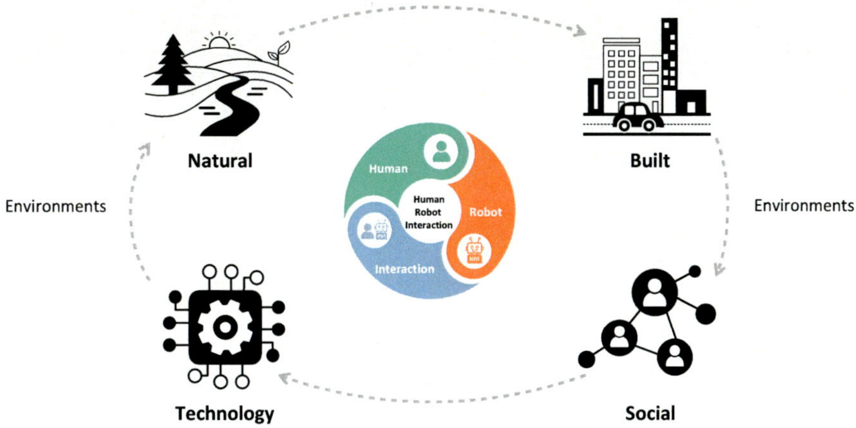

FIGURE 5.1
HRI framework: interaction environments.

Some of the support needs that older adults may have would necessitate a robot's interaction with the natural environment outside of the home. An older adult may need assistance going on a daily neighborhood walk or walking their dog. Another may enjoy hiking as a hobby where an assistive robot would need to be able to traverse more rugged and complex surfaces. Or someone might enjoy gardening as a hobby and need assistance with digging in the ground and handling seeds or plants.

Moreover, including elements of nature in indoor environments promotes health and well-being. Figure 5.2 presents a framework on hypothesized pathways to the mental, physical, social, and behavioral health outcomes from experiences of nature. The framework was used to explore the relationship between the duration, frequency, and intensity of exposure to nature and health in an urban population. The researchers found that people who made long visits to green spaces had lower rates of both depression and high blood pressure. People who visited more frequently had greater social cohesion. Duration and frequency of green space visits were both associated with higher levels of physical activity. Lastly, visits to outdoor green spaces of 30 minutes or more during the course of a week reduced the population prevalence of depression and high blood pressure by up to 7% and 9%, respectively. Given the benefits of people interacting with the natural environment in their everyday lives, robots need to be able to interact with the natural environment as well.

Most early research on mobile robots focused on flat indoor environments, but there is now substantial development in designing robots to traverse complex terrain environments. Robots have been deployed in security and

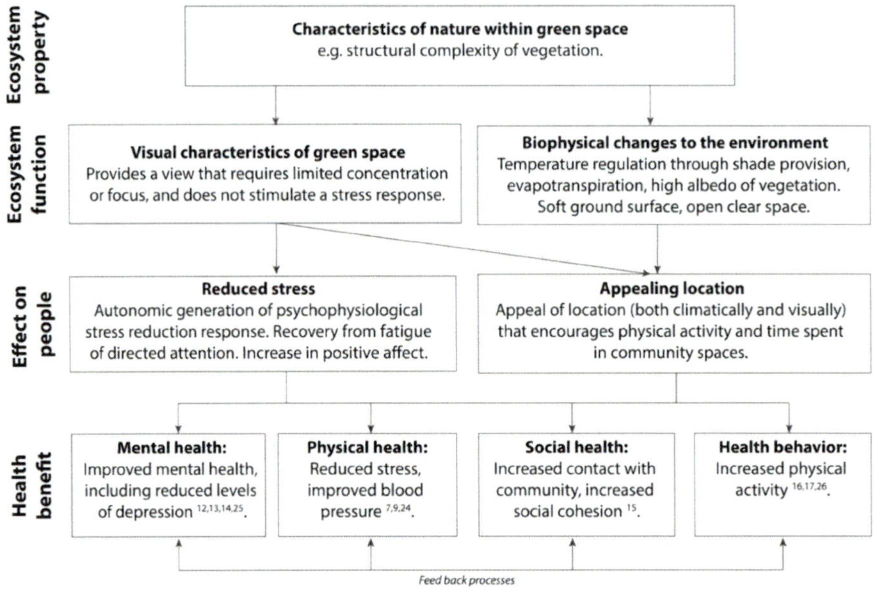

FIGURE 5.2
Hypothesized pathways to the mental, physical, social, and behavioral health outcomes from experiences of nature (from: Shanahan et al., 2016).

search and rescue, field operations, mineral exploration, and deep-space exploration. These robots often have complex adaptive mobility systems, which can adapt to the ground and ensure the robot's stable movement. Robots that can effectively and efficiently traverse a variety of terrain could support older adults in navigating outdoor environments safely. This support could take on a range of formats: a robot could guide a person and warn of possible obstacles, follow a person and hold cargo, monitor their gait for potential fall risk, or physically support a person such as a robotic exoskeleton or a soft robotic device.

The characteristics of the natural environment that should be considered in robot design include:

- Assistance with interests (gardening, birding, wildlife identification)
- Assistance with navigation, walking, and seating
- Interaction with traffic signals, cars, and pedestrians
- Presence of curb cuts
- Surface texture and slope
- Walking speed
- Weather conditions (e.g., rain, snow, extreme heat or cold)
- Need to interact with animals, including indoor pets

5.3 Built

The built environment refers to surroundings that have been created by human activity, such as cities, towns, buildings, transportation infrastructure, and other structures. There are structural differences between private homes, communal living residences, and public environments that have implications for HRI. Environments such as long-term care residences and hospitals are more likely to be compliant with the Americans with Disabilities Act (ADA) accessibility standards and as such having wider hallways and elevators, which would allow for easier autonomous robotic navigation. Other ADA requirements for homes include accessible entrances (e.g., at least one no-step entry), accessible routes (e.g., hallways at least 36 inches wide, smooth, nonslip flooring), bathroom accessibility (e.g., sinks mounted no higher than 34 inches, grab bars around toilets and showers), kitchen accessibility (e.g., countertops no higher than 34 inches), light switches and controls (e.g., positioned between 15 and 48 inches above the floor), stairways and elevators (e.g., handrails on both sides of hallways, elevators or stairlifts for multistory homes). In contrast, private homes vary in size, number of rooms, dimensions of rooms, and number of floors, and likely have stairs. Below we will highlight the built environments most relevant to older adults in greater detail: homes and buildings (i.e., healthcare, wellness, community).

5.3.1 Home

Most older adults live in private homes. Some live with a spouse or other family member(s), and many live alone. Their homes come in a variety of shapes and sizes, but there are standard features that should be considered in robot design including:

- Appliances
- Clutter and other obstacles
- Entrances
- Floor surfaces
- Hallways and doorways
- Lighting
- Multiple stories/stairs, possibly nonstandard (e.g., shallow/deep, short/tall)

The importance of "aging in place" has become a commonplace phrase that is often interpreted as people settling in a home and wanting to age in that home indefinitely. However, we must understand the more nuanced meaning of "place" in this phrase. One aspect is that what people call home can look quite different from person to person, and it is misguided to assume that one version of a home is better or even more common than another. Another nuance is that what a person chooses as their home might change over time. Someone who lives in a large home may choose to downsize as they get older. Someone who lives in a two-story home may choose to move to a single-story home as they age. The crucial meaning of aging in place is that most people would like to age in the particular home and/or community of their choice. In fact, there can be significant fear and opposition to being forced to move from one's choice of a home. Nevertheless, some older adults do move to a different home setting that offers support for present or anticipated support needs. For example, someone who lives in a multistory single-family home may choose to move to a senior living condominium in anticipation future assistance needs or for the available amenities. These types of communities may offer a range of services such as meals and social opportunities as well as educational, arts, and recreational activities. Robot support could enable older adults who live in these communities to remain there longer and reduce their need to hire formal caregivers for tasks such as laundry, cleaning, security, organization, and nutrition. There are a wide range of options for living arrangements including the following:

- Accessory dwelling units (ADUs): Small apartments, sometimes called "in-law suites," may be an addition to a family member's house or a separate home on the property. The popularity of ADUs has increased since the turn of the century.
- Age-restricted communities: At least 80% of the homes in these communities must include one resident aged 55 or older by law. They are often referred to as "active adult communities" and offer amenities such as swimming pools, gyms, and tennis and pickleball courts.
- Senior apartments: Typically, rental units restricted to people aged 55 and older and may include age-friendly features, such as limited grab bars and stairs. Some senior housing is subsidized, enabling residents to qualify for a reduced rent. Some offer meals and other supportive programs such as exercise classes and social opportunities.
- Cohousing communities: These communities may be multigenerational (but not necessarily familial) and typically include joint participation in some activities such as cooking, gardening, and recreation.
- House sharing: A home (rented or purchased) may be shared by friends or strangers to help reduce costs while adding social support and companionship. The housemates may be of similar age but not necessarily. An older adult may rent out a room in their home to a younger person who can provide some care and transportation support in exchange for a reduced rent.
- Naturally occurring retirement community (NORC): Sometimes referred to as a village model. Older adults in a neighborhood

or apartment building may form a group, or even formalize as a nonprofit, to share resources such as transportation, in-home care, and yard work. NORCs can also provide social opportunities.

Although still a less frequent residence choice, a growing number of older adults are moving to some type of long-term care community (e.g., continuing care retirement community [CCRC]) to meet their present or anticipated assistance needs. These communities typically offer meals, cleaning and laundry, and management of chronic conditions. They may be the first to deploy robots for practical reasons (i.e., cost/value). Robots could serve many members of the community who live there while also reducing work demands for the staff by completing physically demanding tasks (e.g., cleaning, lifting). For older adults who have or anticipate needing higher levels of assistance, communal or residential housing options include:

- CCRCs: These communities offer a continuum of care. Residents typically start in independent living, and as their needs dictate, they move to housing with higher levels of care, such as assisted living, memory care, and/or nursing care.
- Assisted living: In these facilities, residents may live in their own room or suite or a shared room. They provide access to clinical care, three meals a day, and medication management. If needed, they can provide assistance with bathing and dressing.
- Group care homes: Group care homes, sometimes referred to as "residential care homes" and "board and care homes," are a type of assisted living community and offer similar services. Residents have a private or shared room. They are state-licensed homes, owned by an individual or a company.
- Memory care: These are specialized care facilities for residents with dementia (e.g., Alzheimer's disease). They are intended to provide structured routines to reduce stress, often have circular hallways to make wayfinding easier, and have locked elevators, front doors, and stairwells to keep residents safe. They may offer activities to stimulate cognition such as singing, reading, and arts and crafts. Memory care units are often a part of CCRCs.
- Nursing homes: These facilities provide 24-hour personal and healthcare for adults who need help with basic activities of living, such as bathing, dressing, eating, using the bathroom, and transferring in and out of beds or chairs.

5.3.2 Buildings

Deploying robots in community buildings provides the opportunity for a single robot to support multiple older adults, again potentially improving the deployment cost-effectiveness. Community buildings where older adults may frequent include those that offer health and wellness services and community participation activities.

Healthcare-related robots include those who assist with surgery, rehabilitation, radiotherapy, and disinfection. Mobility robots are another common type of robot in the healthcare environment, including those that deliver meals, linens, medications, specimens, and supplies. Robots can assist with strenuous tasks such as moving patients, beds, or machines, thereby reducing the likelihood of injury for hospital staff.

Environmental considerations for mobility robots include navigating complex hospital layouts and potential dynamic obstacles such as wheelchairs, beds, stretchers, oxygen tanks, intravenous (IV) poles, and other medical equipment. If a robot is in the wrong place at the wrong time, it could disrupt existing workflows and cause an obstacle itself during a crisis if people and objects are moving very quickly.

Safety is an especially important consideration in healthcare environments, given that robots may be in the presence of or interacting with physically vulnerable people. For robots that interact physically with patients, artificial skin can give medical robots a better sense of touch, including the ability to sense temperature and pressure. This enhanced sensing could improve the safety of the robots. Other considerations include power consumption and energy, maintenance, and platform cybersecurity. The complex and dynamic environment of a healthcare setting can reduce the robot's energy efficiency. The high-use and multiuser context could increase maintenance demands, and the protected health information involved could increase the needs for cybersecurity.

The intricate nature of healthcare robots and the critical stakes involved in this context necessitate deep stakeholder collaboration during development and design. Creating successful healthcare robots requires extensive collaboration among engineers, researchers, medical professionals, patients, and manufacturers.

Robots have potential to support older adults in wellness environments. Although the wellness industry has not seen as much application and innovation in robotics as healthcare contexts, there is great potential for future development. As people are living longer, maintaining health and preventing or managing chronic conditions is becoming more critical. Engaging in exercise can help prevent and manage chronic conditions.

Exercise environments may be open gyms or areas filled with exercise equipment. Areas with large pieces of equipment may not have room to allow for a robot to navigate. Open gyms may have smaller pieces of equipment such as dumbbells, exercise mats, and chairs that may be moved to different locations often – so surfaces and obstacles could vary. Alternatively, robots may be coaching or assisting an older adult in their exercises, such as tai chi. Some of the same considerations are relevant in both healthcare and wellness environments, including safety issues when a robot physically interacts with an older person and the complex and dynamic characteristics of their environments.

An environment in which wellness classes might be offered is that of a senior center in the community. This type of center often offers other activities as well as some services. Activities might include social and recreational (e.g., bingo, bridge, Mah-Jongg, arts and crafts), educational and arts (e.g., musical performances, lectures, plays), and health screenings and education. Services can include transportation as well as meal and nutrition programs. There may be a wide range of spaces in the community center for providing these activities including multiuse rooms (e.g., wellness classes or social, recreational, educational, and arts activities), kitchen and food preparation areas, offices, fitness rooms, and natatoriums. Some centers have technology rooms where seniors can use (and learn to use) computers and other technologies.

Most community buildings will meet ADA accessibility criteria such as wide hallways, automatic doors, and elevators. However, the older adults who occupy them could have a wide range of limitations and abilities, and levels of vulnerability that need to be considered in robot design.

5.3.3 Transportation

A significant challenge for people as they age is transportation. Declines in vision, hearing, cognition, and reflexes can prevent some older adults from driving when they get older as well as increase accident rates for those who do drive. Fatal crash rates also increase for those 75 years of age and older (see Figure 5.3) partly because of increases in frailty rates with older adulthood. Robots such as robot passengers or driving assistants, and autonomous or

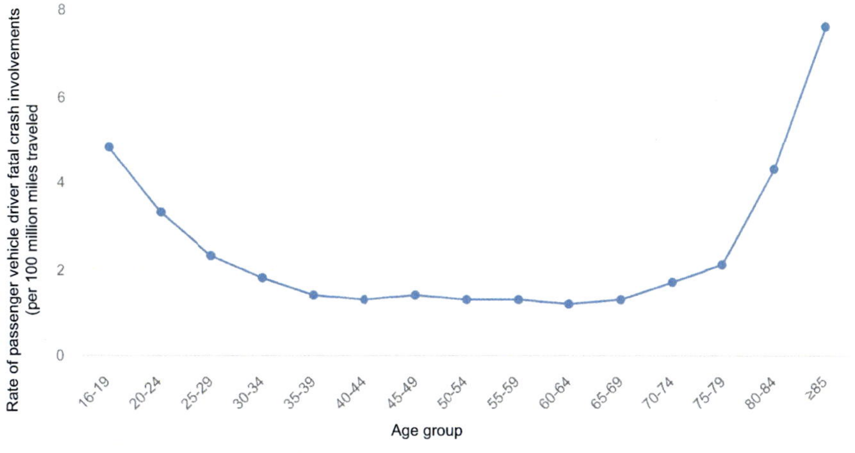

FIGURE 5.3
Passenger vehicle fatal crash involvements per 100 million miles traveled by driver age, April 1, 2016–March 31, 2017 (from: Insurance Institute for Highway Safety, 2020).

semiautonomous vehicles may help to mitigate the growing risk of accidents and of fatal accidents experienced by older adult drivers.

Robotics pose an opportunity to improve transportation for everyone, but older adults may benefit particularly. Table 5.1 presents a range of potential implications of robotics on transportation, as well as examples of impacts and considerations for the aging population. Design and technology advancements needed to drive these transportation innovations include those in autonomous navigation systems, sensor fusion techniques, machine learning, artificial intelligence, HRI, integration of 5G connectivity, edge computing and cloud robotics, multi-robot collaboration, advanced collision avoidance systems, and augmented reality.

TABLE 5.1

Implications and impact of robotics on transportation

Implications	Example Impacts	Considerations for Aging Population
Improved transportation efficiency	Optimized traffic flow, and reducing congestion and travel times. Intelligent routing algorithms and real-time data analysis help to identify efficient routes.	Some older adults may prioritize other factors over efficiency, such as avoiding freeways or dangerous roads.
Enhanced safety	Advanced collision avoidance systems, real-time monitoring, and risks and accident mitigation. Reduced human error, improved response times, and autonomous navigation.	Some older adults, particularly those with frailty, may need different parameters for injury prevention. Age-related changes in abilities such as reaction time, strength, vision, and hearing need to be integrated.
Increased accessibility	Personalized assistance, accessible interfaces, and accommodation of diverse mobility needs, ensuring equitable access to transportation options for individuals with disabilities, aging populations, and those in underserved areas.	Older adults may need assistance with multiple aspects of transportation including planning, timing, routing, transfer into and out of the vehicle, as well as driving.

(Continued)

TABLE 5.1 (Continued)

Urban planning and infrastructure	More efficient transportation systems create more sustainable and livable cities. Optimized road networks, designated lanes for autonomous vehicles, improved public transportation integration.	Older drivers may need additional training and practice when implementing new transportation infrastructure.
Employment and workforce changes	New employment opportunities created in robot maintenance, system monitoring, and data analysis (though possible job displacement in some areas). Critical to support workforce through reskilling and reemployment initiatives.	Some of those older workers will be older adults and may need more in-depth training and practice as they have less technology experience in general.
Social dynamics and user acceptance	Need for increase public attitudes, acceptance, and trust in robotics for transportation. Critical to build public awareness, address concerns, and foster inclusivity design and deployment.	Include older users in the design and deployment process. May need more in-depth training and education about potential benefits for older adults to facilitate acceptance.
Data privacy and security	Robot-assisted mobility systems involve the collection and processing of large amounts of data. Need for ensuring data privacy and security measures, and maintaining public trust (e.g., secure data protocols, encryption techniques, transparent data handling practices).	May need more in-depth training and education about data privacy and security for those with less technology experience.
Social equity and inclusion	Need to ensure accessible to all, including older adults and disadvantaged communities, with reasonable price range.	Include a wide range of older adults, with varying levels of physical and cognitive abilities, at all aspects of design process, and feasibility and usability testing.

Source: Adapted from Usmani et al. (2023).

5.4 Social

The social environment refers to the social and cultural relationships between people. They include family, friendships, caregivers, healthcare providers, and those in the groups people belong to and neighborhoods and communities in which they live. The social environment will vary based on what type of building the robot is located in. In home environments, there may be informal or formal caregivers, or there may be other family members or a roommate. In a senior living environment, there may be several other older adults (e.g., some group care homes) or hundreds (e.g., some CCRCs). In healthcare and wellness buildings, there will likely be many other people in the environment with a variety of roles (e.g., providers, other patients, family members, instructors, coaches, other participants). In community and government buildings, there will likely be many other people with varying roles (e.g., other residents, community leaders, volunteers, government officials, service providers, law enforcement and emergency services providers, administrators).

In many of these settings, there could be multiple users of a robot. The benefit of having multiple users is that it may make the robot more cost-effective. Another benefit of using a robot in a communal environment is that there may be multiple people available to help control and maintain the robot. However, having multiple users creates more complicated programming and interactions for the robot. The robot will need to learn a wide range of assistance needs and preferences.

5.4.1 Care network

Aging in place does not preclude getting assistance. Many older adults require assistance managing chronic conditions (see Figure 2.3) and compensating for disabilities (see Figure 2.4). Hence, older adults may be living in their homes with very little assistance or with substantial assistance from informal and formal caregivers. An individual's care network may include spouses or partners, adult family members, physicians, visiting nurses, health aides, social workers, and physical, occupational, and respiratory therapists.

The characteristics of care networks that should be considered in robot design include:

- Multiple users and different levels of robot access (e.g., full vs. limited).
- Different types of interaction (e.g., physical, in-person, remote, telemedicine, sending/receiving data to/from the robot).
- Variable social dynamics within a family, and information access will need to reflect individual values and preferences.
- Task needs may change from hour to hour or day to day based on the different users.

5.4.2 Culture

The social environment will vary based on demographic variables such as cultural background. Multigenerational households (i.e., family members of multiple generation live in the same home) are more common in some parts of the world and in some cultures (see Figure 5.4). For example, in the United States, multigenerational households are more common in African American, Asian, and Hispanic families. The benefits of multigenerational households include social and emotional support, financial security, home security, and support for age-related needs for assistance with everyday activities. Cognitive and physical health benefits have been associated with older adults living with their adult children or grandchildren. The younger household members can receive benefits in multigenerational households as well, such as childcare support and stronger family bonds.

Although there are benefits to multigenerational households, there are costs that can result from an adult child providing care for their parent, including higher stress, missed days of work, negative economic impacts, psychological distress, and guilt. Robots may be able to reduce these costs and provide respite for adult children caregivers by assisting older adults with some of their needs.

The characteristics of multigenerational households that should be considered in robot design include:

- Possibility of multiple age groups as users including adult children and grandchildren as well as other extended family members.

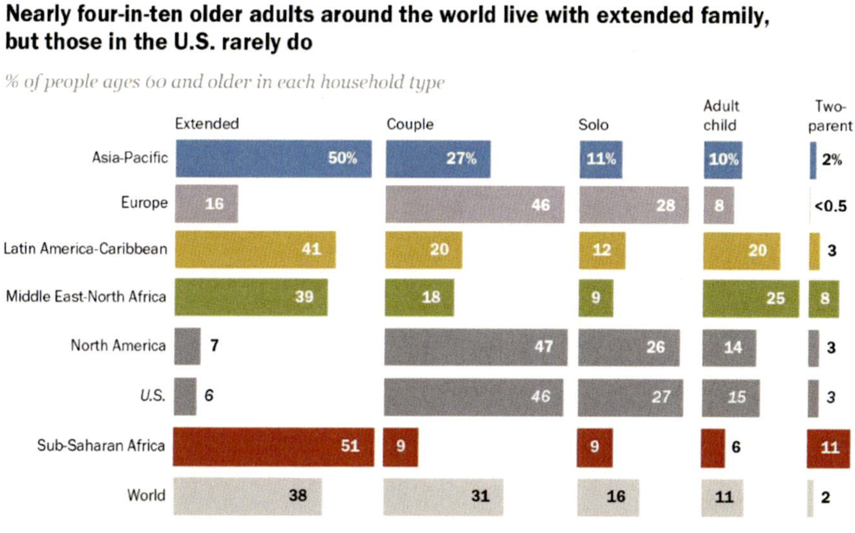

FIGURE 5.4
Percent of people aged 60 and older in each household type (from: Ausubel, 2020).

- In addition to providing assistance to older users, assistance may need to be provided to other users as well, such as support for work for adult children and for learning for grandchildren.
- Possibly greater density in the home: more people to navigate through, and possibly more furniture, etc.

5.5 Technology

The technology environment is defined by the technological infrastructure, hardware, software, and systems that exist in the environment or are connected to the environment (e.g., the cloud). Robots will not be functioning in isolation but rather in a technology ecosystem. Future homes will likely be integrated with smart technology to create living spaces that are more comfortable, efficient, and secure. Appliances and home systems will likely be controlled with support from AI, including lights, temperature, and security. Smart health devices such as scales, pillboxes, and wearable cardiac monitors will be used. Robots will need to be integrated in these smart home and health systems.

Figure 5.5 presents a potential future home technology environment with a variety of health-related devices and robots that would all work together to support the health and well-being of older adults. As depicted, technology will likely be sending and receiving data between different types of robots (e.g., assistive robot, robotic pet), remote caregivers, wearables (e.g., smart patch, fall detection sensor, and a smart watch, socks and shoes), and devices such as smart rugs, monitors, scales, and smart pillboxes.

Much of the storage and integration of data will likely take place in the cloud. AI will be able to personalize an older adult's experience in their home to meet their preferences, such as lighting and temperature. It will be able to learn their habits and consider environmental factors to provide predictive automation. It will also be able to have contextual awareness and identify functional declines and assistance needs of older adults in real time. AI will likely be integrated into many different technologies around the home.

Ideally, all of these technologies would create a cohesive and automated home environment, providing safety and cost-saving benefits, as well as convenience benefits. For example, home automation systems could alert a robot if any motion is detected in a home when an older adult is asleep, and the robot could wake them up and call the appropriate authority in the event of a dangerous situation. Or a smart door lock could identify that a door was left open and the robot could close it and lock it, preventing an intruder and heat or cooling loss.

However, there will need to be interoperability between all of the technologies for seamless integration because they may have a variety of

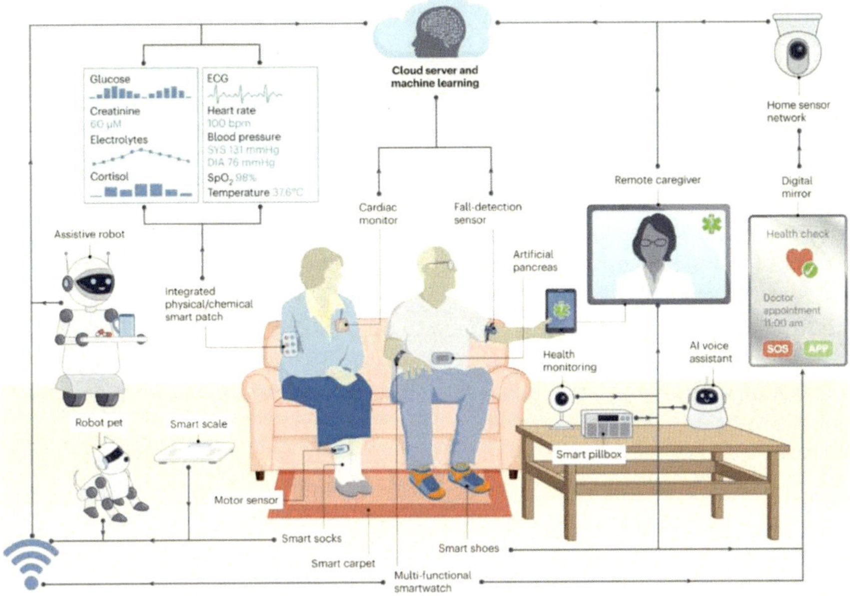

FIGURE 5.5
The future of geriatric healthcare in the home setting (from: Chen et al., 2023).

manufacturers. If not, they will be unable to communicate or coordinate with one another and could create more difficulties than benefits, or worse, they could cause dangerous situations (e.g., if a robot that provides insulin injections misinterpreted the data coming from a blood glucose monitor). There will also need to be a main point of control for all of the technologies in the home. A robot might be the central organizing system and interface for the human to control such a smart home. In that respect, robots could be at the center of the technology ecosystem in future homes.

If the robots do become the central interface of a home's technology ecosystem, then much more work will need to be done to ensure that older adults can easily use them to control their smart homes. They will need to be able to complete basic operations as well as customize the automation to meet their needs and preferences. They will also need intuitive feedback mechanisms to understand the status of the technology environment.

The larger technology infrastructure should be considered as well. Many technologies including robots are wireless systems that require strong Wi-Fi coverage and broadband service throughout a home or building. Unfortunately, a digital divide still remains in the United States and in other high-income countries. Cost is part of the issue; for some, including many older adults who live on a fixed income, broadband is not affordable. There is also limited high-speed broadband coverage in some low-income neighborhoods, rural areas, and tribal lands.

With the benefits of all of the technologies in the environment comes risk. Security risks and functionality glitches will likely continue as the number of technologies (from different manufacturers) in homes and buildings increases. The sharing of data between users and devices only increases these risks. Older adults are often targeted by technology scams, phishing, and malware, and are more likely to also fall victim to these malicious activities, especially if they have less technology experience. Adults in the working world now may receive training on identifying malicious technology behaviors, but most older adults have not been privy to this information. A crucial part of providing robotic support for older adults is empowering them with information about how to protect their security and privacy when using them in the technology ecosystem.

The characteristics of the technology environment that should be considered in robot design include:

- Technologies may be programmed and managed by a remote care partner or family member
- Likely a mix of new "smart" appliances and lighting and older traditional ones
- Software compatibility and interoperability
- Wi-Fi coverage and strength

5.6 Design guidelines for interaction environments

- Consider a wide range of environments in which older adults may be interacting with robots (i.e., most older adults are not confined to their homes):
  - Natural (e.g., sidewalks as well as rugged terrain)
  - Built (e.g., different types of homes; community centers; healthcare, wellness, and government buildings; transportation)
  - Social (e.g., care network, friends, family)
  - Technology (e.g., smart appliances, health devices)
- Ensure robots can navigate around possible clutter and other obstacles including pets, children, and mobility devices.
- Conduct early testing and deployment of robots in communal living settings to get feedback from a range of users.
- Make sure older adults who are physically frail can interact with the robots safely, especially in healthcare environments.

- Use immersive participatory design to understand the complex and dynamic environments of some users, particularly those with high support needs (see Chapter 8).
- Consider robots in a range of roles and contexts in transportation systems (e.g., as driver or passenger; using private vehicle or public transportation).
- Minimize barriers for older adults to use robotic transportation systems, personal vehicles, as well as public systems.
- Ensure transportation systems consider older adults' unique abilities and limitations, as well as increased injury-protection needs.
- Include multiple stakeholders from the social environment in testing, to maximize ease of use and usefulness for different users.
- Consider cultural representation in early development to ensure norms about aging, caregiving, and living situations are understood.
- If older adults are programming and managing the home technology systems, they may need additional training and technical support (e.g., use, customization, security).
- Include other parts of the technology ecosystem to ensure robots can efficiently and effectively integrate with other technologies.

Recommended readings and links

Readings

Avioz-Sarig, O., Olatunji, S., Sarne-Fleischmann, V., & Edan, Y. (2021). Robotic system for physical training of older adults. *International Journal of Social Robotics 13*, 1109–1124. https://doi.org/10.1007/s12369-020-00697-y

Chen, C., Ding, S., & Wang, J. (2023). Digital health for aging populations. *Nature Medicine, 29*(7), 1623–1630. https://doi.org/10.1038/s41591-023-02391-8

Li, S., Milligan, K., Blythe, P., Zhang, Y., Edwards, S., Palmarini, N., Corner, L., Ji, Y., Zhang, F., & Namdeo, A. (2023). Exploring the role of human-following robots in supporting the mobility and wellbeing of older people. *Scientific Reports, 13*(1), 6512. https://doi.org/10.1038/s41598-023-33837-1

Mitzner, T. L., Chen, T. L., Kemp, C. C., & Rogers, W. A. (2014). Identifying the potential for robotics to assist older adults in different living environments. *International Journal of Social Robotics, 6*(2), 213–227. https://doi.org/10.1007/s12369-013-0218-7

Nagasawa, T., Oyake, K., Kawahara, M., Kaneko, S.-I., & Capi, G. (2022). Development of a walking assistive robot for elderly people in outdoor environments. *2nd International Conference on Image Processing and Robotics (ICIPRob)*, Colombo, Sri Lanka (pp. 1–5). https://doi.org/10.1109/ICIPRob54042.2022.9798726

Nakagawa, Y., Park, K., Ueda, H., & Ono, H. (2014). Driving assistance with conversation robot for elderly drivers. In C. Stephanidis & M. Antona (Eds.) *Universal access in human-computer interaction. Aging and assistive environments. UAHCI 2014. Lecture notes in computer science* (vol. 8515). Heraklion. https://doi.org/10.1007/978-3-319-07446-7_71

Usmani, U. A., Happonen, A., & Watada, J. (2023). Revolutionizing transportation: Advancements in robot-assisted mobility systems. In M. Tuba, S. Akashe, & A. Joshi (Eds.) *ICT Infrastructure and Computing. ICT4SD 2023. Lecture notes in networks and systems* (vol. 754). Goa. https://doi.org/10.1007/978-981-99-4932-8_55

Wilson, C. M., Boright, L., Louie, W. G., Shahverdi, P., Arena, S. K., Benbow, R., Wilson, J. R., Chen, Q., Rousso, K., & Huang, N. (2023). Effect of robotic delivery of physical activity and fall prevention exercise in older adults: A pilot cohort study. *Cureus, 15*(8), e44264. https://doi.org/10.7759/cureus.44264

Zhao, Q., Chen, Z., Landis, C. D., Lytle, A., Rao, A. K., Zanotto, D., & Guo, Y. (2022). Gait monitoring for older adults during guided walking: An integrated assistive robot and wearable sensor approach. *Wearable Technologies, 3*, e28. https://doi.org/10.1017/wtc.2022.23

Links

A robotic helping hand for aging in place:
https://betterworld.mit.edu/spectrum/issues/2023-spring/a-robotic-helping-hand-for-aging-in-place/

Can robots save nursing homes?
https://www.nytimes.com/2022/04/21/realestate/nursing-home-robots.html

Co-designing with older adults, for older adults: Robots to promote physical activity:
https://intuitivecomputing.github.io/publications/2023-hri-antony.pdf

Human-following robots have potential to promote healthy aging:
https://medicalxpress.com/news/2023-08-human-following-robots-potential-healthy-aging.html

Japanese automakers look to robots to aid the elderly:
https://www.scientificamerican.com/article/japanese-automakers-look-to-robots-to-aid-the-elderly/

Moxi delivery robot at MacNeal Hospital:
https://www.youtube.com/watch?v=iGxz2dVorvc

Older people are more likely to live alone in the U.S. than elsewhere in the world:
https://www.pewresearch.org/short-reads/2020/03/10/older-people-are-more-likely-to-live-alone-in-the-u-s-than-elsewhere-in-the-world/

Robotic shorts support people when walking:
https://www.sciencedaily.com/releases/2024/11/241114125854.htm#

6

Ethical considerations

6.1 Overview of ethical considerations

One challenge that older adults with cognitive impairments experience is face-name recognition. What if an older person had a personal robot that would recognize someone approaching them and tell them who it was? This might be wonderful for the older person in terms of reducing their stress and supporting their social interactions. But what about the invasion of privacy for the other person and the need to store faces of acquaintances for the matching process?

Or consider an assistive robot for the home that prepares food, does housework, and provides medication reminders. Again, perhaps wonderful for the older adult because it enables them to remain at home with that support. But what if an unintended consequence is that no other humans visit the home for longer periods of time, given that their services are not needed? Would it be better to not have the robot at all?

A home might contain multiple robots that are social, assistive, and mobile, and with sensors that gather vast quantities of data every day. Such data might include the ambient temperature in the home; if the stove has been used; the person's heart rate, sleep quality, food intake, and urine output; the number of people who visited the home in a given week; how many hours the television was on; and so on. Where do the data go? To family members? Insurance companies? Technology developers? Policymakers? Law enforcement? Landlords? The list is seemingly endless.

These are just a few of the myriad ethical issues that surround the field of human–robot interaction (HRI) for older adults. How should designers, family members, policymakers, healthcare providers, and other stakeholders ensure that they are making ethical decisions? It starts with thinking about the issues, the range of users, use contexts, potential consequences as well as potential unintended consequences. Many of the considerations are not unique to robots. However, the fact that robots can be mobile or sociable might lead to an exacerbation of ethical considerations.

Likewise, ethical considerations about robots are not specific to older adults. However, they may be more concerned about loss of autonomy, more

DOI: 10.1201/9781032656649-6

susceptible to deception, or more likely to have physical, perceptual, or cognitive needs that increase their reliance on robot support. Consequently, older adults may be more at risk.

6.2 Robot laws and roboethics

Let's start with the classic: Asimov's laws (see Figure 6.1). In the March 1942 issue of *Astounding Science Fiction*, Isaac Asimov published a short story called "Runaround" that was later republished in his short story collection *I, Robot* (Asimov, 1950). The laws conveyed the rules according to which robots should be programmed to protect the humans around them. Fundamental was the idea that robots could not injure humans. Asimov would return to these rules in later stories, expanding on them, and exploring their limits. In 1985, he added the fourth law of robotics in his story "Robots and Empire" (Asimov, 1985), but he called it the Zeroth law, to indicate that it should precede the others: *a robot may not harm humanity or allow humanity to come to harm through inaction*.

Asimov's original *I, Robot* book has been reprinted many times. Figure 6.1 portrays changing media representations over the years with a sampling of the book covers. The original 1950 edition shows the robot carrying a human, presumably saving the person's life, whereas the 2013 edition depicts a profile

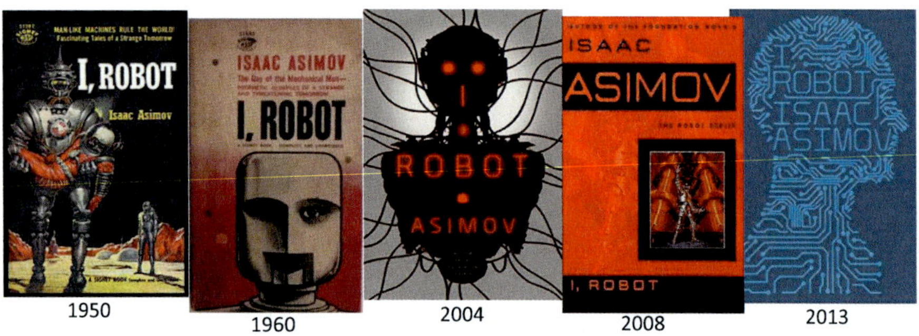

First Law
A robot may not injure a human being, or, through inaction, allow a human being to come to harm.

Second Law
A robot must obey the orders given it by human beings except where such orders would conflict with the First Law.

Third Law
A robot must protect its own existence as long as such protection does not conflict with the First or Second Law.

FIGURE 6.1
Asimov's robot laws (from: Asimov, 1950).

that could be at the head of a human or a humanoid. There were a variety of depictions in between; we present just a small sampling. The rationale (and marketing decisions) behind the different covers is unknown, but the array illustrates how the same content can be packaged in different ways that presumably will influence the readers' views.

On the surface, Asimov's laws may seem straightforward, but once specific situations are considered, their complexity emerges. What if there are multiple humans? Who determines what is harmful? For example, harm to an older adult could be physical, but we should also think about emotional harm. Consider a robot that is programmed to stop a person with dementia from wandering outside and getting lost – a potentially dangerous situation. But, as a result of the robot protecting them from danger, the person ends up being confined indoors, which could cause them emotional distress. Thinking about these ethical issues might result in a different type of robot – one that can accompany the person wherever they go, protect them, and guide them back to their residence – all without constraining their freedom of movement.

Asimov's laws have served as the starting point for numerous discussions about the ethics of robots. They began in the realm of science fiction, but technology advancements have yielded a wide variety of robots with which humans can interact (see Chapter 3), necessitating their careful consideration outside of fictional worlds and into real worlds.

In 2004, there was a conference held on roboethics followed by a workshop in 2006 that led to the Roboethics Roadmap (as described in Veruggio, 2006). Roboethics is a branch of applied ethics that focuses on designing, developing, and using robots. The issues addressed vary broadly, as illustrated by a sampling of chapter titles in *Robot Ethics: The Ethical and Social Implications of Robotics* (Lin et al., 2012):

- Current trends in robotics: Technology and ethics (Bekey)
- Robotics, ethical theory, and metaethics: A guide for the perplexed (Abney)
- Moral machines: Contradiction in terms or abdication of human responsibility (Allen & Wallach)
- Compassionate AI and selfless robotics: A Buddhist approach (Hughes)
- Robots and privacy (Calo)
- Robot caregivers: Ethical issues across the human lifespan (Borenstein & Pearson)
- The rights and wrongs of robot care (Sharkey & Sharkey)
- Roboethics: The applied ethics for a new science (Veruggio & Abney)

An in-depth evaluation of all these topics is beyond the scope of this chapter. However, we want to emphasize the importance of having a technology

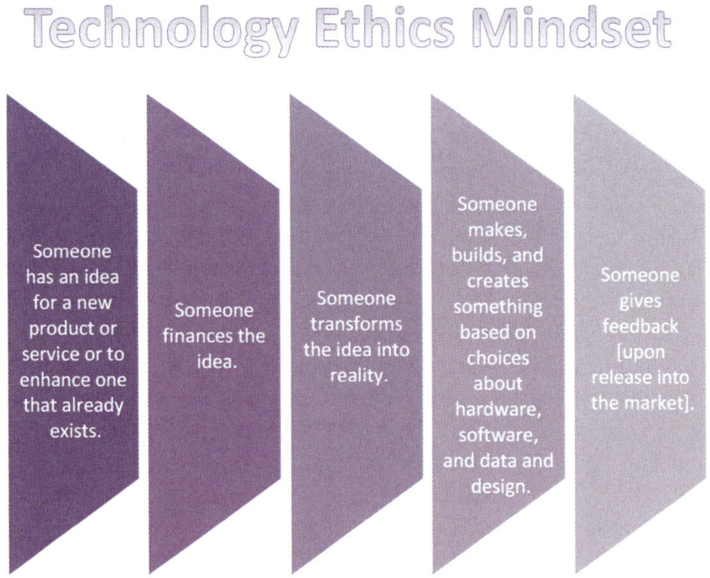

FIGURE 6.2
When to think about ethics (based on Hare, 2021, p. 77).

ethics mindset and considering ethical issues early and throughout the development process and implementation cycle, as depicted in Figure 6.2. Henceforth, we review ethical issues related to robots that might be particularly relevant to older adults.

6.3 Robot care providers

Throughout the book, we have provided examples of the potential for robots to provide care and support for older adults with everyday tasks as well as specifically in healthcare contexts. Despite the potential for robots to increase autonomy by enabling older adults to perform various tasks with robot assistance, this concept raises ethical considerations.

Robots intended to provide care often fall into the category of social assistive robots. There is a growing literature on the ethical issues that will need to be considered in this realm. Figure 6.3 illustrates the distribution of topics from a recent literature review, organized by three general themes:

- *Well-being: Considerations about the person receiving the care.* This theme was the most observed in the literature reviewed. Topics included privacy, security, deception, autonomy, loss of human contact, safety, dignity, emotional attachment, objectification, and morality, among others.

- *Care: The nature of the care being provided and care practices.* Topics included how robots were introduced and integrated into the health-care system, quality of care, influence on humans and their morals, trust, and the impact on care and on care workers.
- *Justice: Societal issues.* The topics in this theme pertained to equity and equality across society members; benefits and costs; economic, political, and ideological considerations; responsibility and assistive practices; and sustainability issues.

The distribution of the themes does not necessarily reflect their importance but represents the state of the science for this broad topic. Certainly, the ethical issues that relate to the person are critically important, but the issues at the level of care practices and justice are important as well, but as yet understudied.

The ethical domains for care robots are elaborated further in Table 6.1. Koh et al. (2023) focused specifically on the potential of pet robots, although the domains listed transcend that specific robot category. The repeated theme in the list is "impact." What is the impact on the care recipient if robots are being used to provide care? Through interviews with care professionals and organizational leaders from different nursing homes they identified individual-level issues (e.g., the importance of aligning pet robots with residents' preferences, individual differences), organization-level issues (e.g., need for alignment with the existing care routines in the nursing home, staff burden), and society-level issues (e.g., cost, regulatory rules).

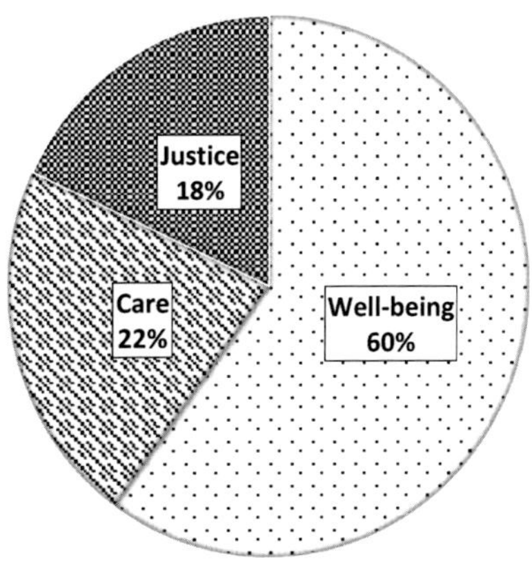

FIGURE 6.3
Ethical issues for social assistive robots (SARs) explored in the literature (from: Boada et al., 2021).

TABLE 6.1

Ethical domains relating to the use of care robots

Ethical Domains	Brief Description
1. Respect for autonomy and privacy	Impact of care robots on the autonomy and privacy of older adults and their care partners.
2. Dignity, objectification, and deception	Impact of care robots on the dignity of older adults, since machines cannot recognize them as persons. This could lead to feelings of objectification. Deception can occur when robots are designed to resemble living beings and become perceived as such.
3. Replacement	Perceiving and regarding care robots as replacements for human caregivers.
4. Social isolation and loneliness	The potential impact of care robots on older adults' feelings of loneliness and social isolation; however, there could be potential negative impacts.
5. Safety, and physical and psychological harm	Potential of physical and psychological harm relating to the use of pet robots, such as distress.
6. Social justice	Equal access and fair distribution of care robots, and the legal responsibility relating to their use.
7. Conceptions of care	Impact of the use of care robots on the societal, organizational, and individual conceptions of what aged care entails and means. The societal values relating to the use of care robots for older people, such as the values of care provision.

Source: From Koh et al. (2023).

Designers should be aware of the range of issues that relate to care robots. The point of ethical considerations is just that – consideration. Be aware of the topics that are relevant to the context of design, explore the potential implications of introducing a robot into that setting, and make concerted efforts to address the issues in the design and deployment of robots that will be supporting the care of people. The goal is to think about how a robot can augment care, not replace the human in the care system, and to determine how robots balance efficiency in care with the preservation of human dignity.

6.4 Safety/risk of harm and consequences

Our HRI framework depicts different types of engagement (see Chapter 4 for details) that can represent situations wherein a robot might potentially harm a human. For example, the robot might be in close proximity to people or perhaps even need to come into physical contact with them, for example, when handing them an item, carrying out a health-related task (e.g., checking blood pressure), or assisting them to stand up from a seated position. These tasks might be very useful for an older adult, but the safety issues need to be carefully considered. Older adults often are at greater risk for falls, and even a minor bump from a robot might throw off their balance (and the consequences of falls can be very serious, such as a broken bone or a traumatic brain injury). Older adults' skin is more fragile, and they may bruise more easily, which needs to be considered for tasks that require physical contact.

A risk assessment should be conducted to identify known safety hazards and determine how best to address them for different users and use contexts. During technical and user testing, potential risks should be identified and addressed. Classic human factors principles with respect to hazards are to (1) design it out, (2) guard against it, or lastly, (3) provide a warning. A simplistic example would be that a robot that will be touching a person should be designed with soft materials. If sharp edges are needed for aspects of the robot, they should be covered in some way so that the person does not come into contact with them. If a hazard cannot be designed out or guarded against, users should be warned about the potential risk and how best to avoid it. For example, users might be told that another person should always be present when the robot is performing a certain task. A run-stop button could be available that would immediately stop the movement of the robot, or a voice command could be programmed and shared with the users.

The primary point is to do an evaluation and carefully consider a wide range of possible risks. A standard approach is to conduct a failure mode and effects analysis, which emerged from reliability engineering. The idea is to review the different components of the system or product – in this case the robot – to identify potential failure modes, their causes, and their effects. Sometimes, a criticality analysis is part of the evaluation as well, wherein the different potential failures are ranked in terms of their criticality. The results of this systematic approach can guide design and production decisions.

A parallel analysis should be conducted from the user side. What types of errors might they make? How might they use the robot in a way that was not intended? Are there circumstances under which they would give an incorrect/inappropriate command that could result in the robot doing something unexpected? Whenever there is a human in the loop of an interaction, human behavior must be considered, and that includes identifying situations where the person might make an error. Errors can be classified as a slip (they did something unintended), a lapse (they forgot to do something), or a mistake (their plan was not appropriate for the situation.)

The ethical issue here is the need to understand the complexity of potential situations and the range of actions that the robot and/or the human might do. These evaluations of robot behavior, human behavior, interaction contexts, potential errors, and consequences will all take time (and often money). However, they must be part of the process, as depicted in Figure 6.2.

An idea to improve understanding, awareness, and solutions for safety issues has been proposed by Major and Shah (2020), which is to develop a "Robot Safety Reporting System." This system would be modeled after approaches in aviation and healthcare wherein accidents as well as near misses can be shared to help avoid similar safety issues by others. Designers could share their collective experiences and challenges to identify trends that could subsequently be corrected and avoided. As robots become more prevalent, this system could enable anonymous reporting by all stakeholders. These data could inform designers as well as policymakers and standards developers. Such a widespread system is not yet in place, but roboticists are developing communities of practice and online forums wherein they share their experiences.

Discussion of safety and risk in the context of robots often focuses primarily on physical issues. However, equally important are emotional and mental health risks. Does the presence of a robot lead to fewer than desired human interactions? There may be unintended consequences of having a robot deliver drinks to a person by reducing opportunities for casual touch or conversation. Is there a risk for older adults with diminished capacity to become emotionally attached to robots (in which case there would be harmful effects if the robot malfunctioned or was taken away from them for some reason). Moreover, robot actions that are appropriate for certain contexts and cultures may be highly inappropriate for other contexts and cultures, thereby making individuals uncomfortable.

6.5 Privacy and security

Privacy and security are distinct concepts, but they are often discussed together. They both relate to the management and protection of personal information. Privacy and security concerns may influence an older adult's or a care partner's willingness to have a robot in their home. Privacy relates to the person's control over their personal information and how it gets shared with others, especially sensitive information. Security relates to ensuring that the information is only shared the way they want it to be shared (i.e., the information cannot be hacked). For example, consider a robot with cameras – the privacy issue relates to knowing (and controlling) who can view the information through the cameras, when the cameras are turned on, how the information is being stored, and who it is shared with. Security issues relate to the assurance that private information is stored and shared in such a way that people without viewing privileges are unable to view it (via password protection, encryption, intranet storage only, or other established methods).

Tolerance related to privacy and security issues is very personal. Some people are more open and willing to share information, whereas others may not want anyone to know what goes on in their lives. Such tolerance levels may change over time, for example, as needs for support increase. An older adult may be willing to give up some privacy if it means that they can remain living in a preferred location. How do privacy issues change from an individual home environment to a congregate living environment or to public spaces?

The robot could provide privacy protection. Consider a robot shower, for example. Rather than having a human assist with showering, a person might prefer a robot to assist, thereby enabling them to shower alone and preserve their dignity – likewise with other personal tasks such as hygiene, dressing, or toileting. The ability, or lack thereof, to perform these tasks independently is often predictive of the need to move into residential care facilities or to require home healthcare assistance. A robot might be able to both provide support and privacy to an individual and preserve their autonomy.

Ethical issues arise especially if older adults are unable to make decisions for themselves or when it is not clear to them exactly what the privacy and security risks are. With respect to cameras, for example, the user must understand when cameras are on, where the information is being transmitted or stored, and who will have viewing privileges. In addition, robots can be gathering a lot of other information via sensors that can capture activities, behavior patterns, visitors, biometric information, and so on. How can these technological activities be presented in a way that the older user can make informed decisions?

Consider a telehealth robot that is placed in the home of an older adult to be used while they are recovering from spine surgery and completing their rehabilitation. Who is responsible for ensuring that the privacy and security wishes of the patient (and anyone else in the home) are protected? All these entities could have some responsibility:

- The patient
- Family members
- Robotics company
- Healthcare provider
- Hospital administrator
- Insurance company
- Government regulators
- Standards developers

This example illustrates the complexity of the ethical issues that will arise as robots become more widespread. What happens if the robot malfunctions? Who is responsible if there is a security breach? What happens if the patient or someone else in the home gets injured? These are complex issues that do not have easy answers, but that must be considered as we progress in this field.

6.6 Design guidelines for ethics

- Clearly define the problem, the solution, and the relevant stakeholders who might be affected by the introduction of a robot.
- Review ethical topics to identify which ones might be relevant for a particular HRI situation.
- Explore different dimensions of situations and perspectives of various stakeholders.
- Develop priorities to guide decision-making (e.g., maximize autonomy of the person, minimize harm).
- Consider the consequences of different design decisions.
- Ensure transparency of robot decisions and actions so the human understands the reasons.
- Conduct failure mode and effects analysis for the robot and human error analysis for the person to identify – and mitigate – safety risks.
- Attend to physical safety risks as well as emotional and mental health risks.
- Iteratively review potential ethical issues at different stages (idea conception à market introduction).
- Consider ethical issues related to well-being, care practices, and justice.

Recommended readings and links

Readings

Asimov, I. (1950). *I, Robot*. Doubleday.

Asimov, I. (1985). *Robots and empire*. Grafton.

Boada, J. P., Maestre, B. R., & Genís, C. T. (2021). The ethical issues of social assistive robotics: A critical literature review. *Technology in Society*, *67*, 101726. https://doi.org/10.1016/j.techsoc.2021.101726

Hare, S. (2021). *Technology is not neutral: A short guide to technology ethics*. London Publishing Partnership.

Lin, P., Abney, K., & Bekey, G. (2012). *The ethical and social implications of robots*. MIT Press.

Major, L., & Shah, J. (2020). *What to expect when you're expecting robots*. Basic Books.

Mitzner, T. L., Chen, T. L., Kemp, C. C., & Rogers, W. A. (2014). Identifying the potential for robotics to assist older adults in different living environments. *International Journal of Social Robotics*, *6*(2), 213–227.

Sharit, J. (2012). Human error and human reliability analysis. In G. Salvendy (Ed.), *Handbook of human factors and ergonomics* (4th ed., pp. 734–800). Wiley & Sons.

Links

Association for Advancing Automation: Robot ethics: Where values and engineering meet:
https://www.automate.org/robotics/blogs/robot-ethics-where-values-and-engineering-meet

Guidance for performing failure mode and effects analysis with performance improvement projects:
www.cms.gov/medicare/provider-enrollment-and-certification/qapi/downloads/guidanceforfmea.pdf

7

HRI design methods and assessment measures

7.1 Overview of human–robot interaction design methods and assessment measures

Need-driven design refers to a design thinking approach focused on the real needs of the potential users of a technology. This approach is critical for ensuring robots will be useful and usable, and therefore more likely to be adopted by users. When considering older adults as robot users, that means understanding their needs (and preferences; see Chapters 2 and 4) for robotic support. Given that most workers in the technology and robotics industry are younger adults, careful attention needs to be given to understanding the older adult users' needs. Otherwise, designers could rely on assumed needs that may be based on negative deficit-based stereotypes of aging or on anecdotal experiences from people they know. Moreover, including older adults in the design process will likely improve the usability for all ages.

Imagine a scenario with a robot designed to assist older adults. The robot developer assumes that the adult children of older adults will be their primary consumer. Because of that assumption, they focus on researching the adult children's needs and preferences for how the robot will assist their parent. An adult child might purchase the robot, but that does not mean it will be adopted by their parent. Rather it might just become like a piece of furniture in their home. The primary user (in this case an older adult) must be prioritized in acceptance and usability research. Other stakeholders can be included as well but not to the exclusion of the older end user. In this chapter, we provide direction for including older adults in the design process by discussing relevant design methods as well as assessment measures.

7.2 Design methods

Below we describe a variety of design methods that can be used to evaluate a wide range of human–robot interaction (HRI) issues. The methods

DOI: 10.1201/9781032656649-7

highlight the importance of engaging older adults in research, including those with different abilities and disabilities. Personas can be useful particularly in early stages of design, when identifying robot features that can support tasks and environments. Participatory design methods can be even more impactful and would be an optimal next step after developing initial prototypes with personas. Target end users, when included in the design process, can provide specific feedback and redirection to designers. Involving older adults in research studies during robot development can provide important insights into design as well. When doing so, researchers can use a variety of approaches for demonstrating robot capabilities including showing videos that demonstrate a robot's functionality as well as Wizard of Oz experiments (see the "Demonstrating robot capabilities" section for more information about Wizard of Oz experiments). They can use a variety of research methods including questionnaires; surveys; individual and focus group interviews; and observation, interaction, simulation, and single case studies. Depending on the timing of the research, formative (early in the design process) and/or summative (after a prototype has been developed) evaluations may be used. The research may take place in controlled laboratory environments, in virtual environments, or in natural, real-world contexts. Users may be older adults with typical age-related changes or older adults from specific populations (e.g., mild cognitive impairment, physical disabilities, vision impairments).

7.2.1 Including people with different abilities and disabilities

The number of older adults with varying abilities and disabilities is growing. More and more people are aging with diagnoses that may affect their abilities, such as Parkinson's disease, mild cognitive impairment, or dementia. Disabilities such as mobility, vision, and hearing also increase with age. Lack of participation of people with different abilities and disabilities in research can be the result of issues such as lack of awareness of those populations, rigid inclusion criteria, transportation barriers, and inaccessible research facilities and materials. Excluding these people from research studies may bring the external validity of those studies into question, particularly given the growing prevalence of the number of persons aging with different abilities and disabilities in the general population. By including these groups, researchers can increase adoption and generalizability of their findings, as well as better serve and support diverse populations.

We have developed guidelines for including older adults in general, as well as those with hearing, vision, and mobility disabilities in research (see Bayles et al., 2021; see links at the end of this chapter). The guidelines focus on designing study materials that are accessible, developing recruitment and screening strategies to reach these populations, and making the testing experience and environment more accessible, comfortable, and safe.

7.2.2 Personas

Personas are fictional people created by using actual research data about a population or, in the case of designing a robot, a user group (see Figure 7.1 for example persona). They can be created from compiled data from multiple people from a particular population or based on data from an individual representative of that population. For example, the persona in Figure 7.1 was developed based on interviews and observations with multiple older adults living independently with mobility disabilities. Personas are a valuable tool in user-centered design. They provide rich details about the target user group in terms of their specific needs, goals, preferences, and everyday activities and behaviors. They can illustrate the diversity of users in terms of sex, age, race, culture, and other person characteristics that should be considering in the design process (see Chapter 2). They evoke an empathic experience for designers, allowing them to have insights into the users' perspectives. They make the context concrete to support consideration of ethical issues. In these ways, personas can help robot designers make more informed decisions about robot design elements, features, functions, and implementation potential.

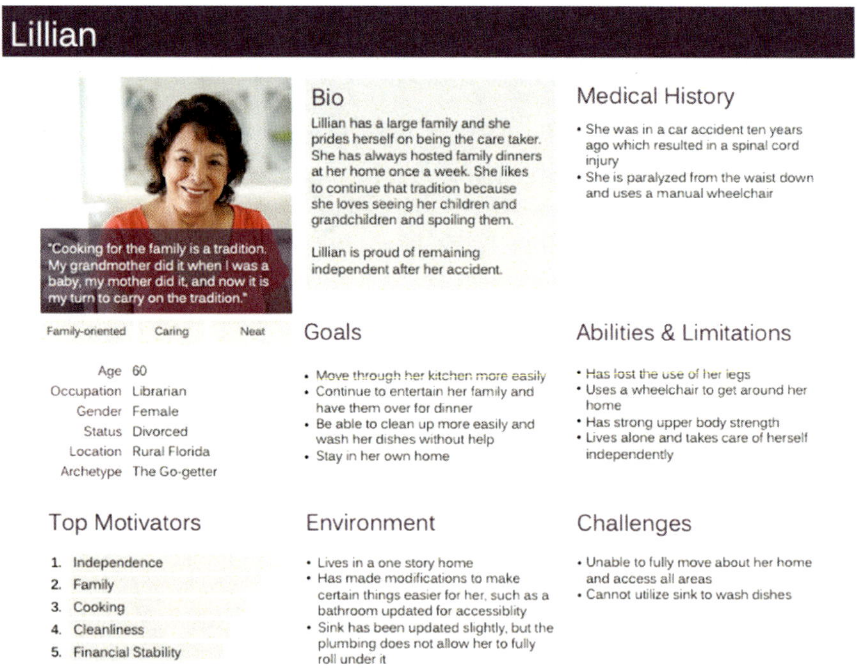

FIGURE 7.1
Example persona of an adult aging with a mobility disability (from: TechSAge Tool: Personas for Designing for Individuals Aging with Mobility Impairment https://techsage.gatech.edu/sites/default/files/2021-01/Design%20Personas%20TS%20Tool_0.pdf).

One caveat to the use of personas for design is that they can be limiting if they are not representative of the target user group. For a heterogeneous group – such as older adults – it may be worthwhile to develop multiple personas that will illustrate the range of potential needs that should be considered in the design process. Such an approach might help to broaden their thinking of the designers.

7.2.3 Participatory design

Participatory design can be generally defined as a collaborative design process that actively involves end users, stakeholders, and designers in product development. This process capitalizes on the experiences, capabilities, limitations, and preferences of end users and other stakeholders to create a more useful and usable product.

During the participatory design process, a range of methods may be used, including quantitative, qualitative, and ethnographic approaches, as well as concept generation and co-design activities. These methods include card sorting, story boarding, drawing/sketching, interviews, focus groups, and workshops (see Figure 7.2 for an example of participatory design in HRI research with older adults). Workshops are the most frequently used method when conducting HRI participatory design research with older adults, which enables multiple methods to be incorporated. For a workshop format, the number of participants in a session would typically be less than 10, at least 2–4 of whom would be representative users. Depending on the purpose, there may be participants from the technology development side, such as a designer or engineer, and/or someone from business or marketing. There would also be a facilitator for the session.

The amount or level of participation of a stakeholder can vary depending on the design goals. Sometimes the term *co-creation* is used in participatory design, which refers generally to collaboration between diverse stakeholders at all project stages, from defining the problem to the final stages of the project. The co-creation principle encompasses co-design and co-production. In co-design the stakeholders are involved in designing solutions to a prespecified problem, whereas in co-production stakeholders are only involved in the implementation of a previously developed solution or product for a previously agreed upon problem (i.e., the focus is on how to allocate resources and assets within these parameters).

Immersive participatory design can be thought of as maximizing the participatory design principle. It involves conducting research or testing in the users' environment where the users, other stakeholders, and researchers are all significantly engaged in the design process. This immersive experience provides deeper insight into the complexities and constraints in the users' environment. Chapter 8 describes an example of our work using immersive participatory design in the development of robotics to support people who are aging with significant disabilities (see Figure 8.6 for an example of a robotics product resulting from immersive participatory design).

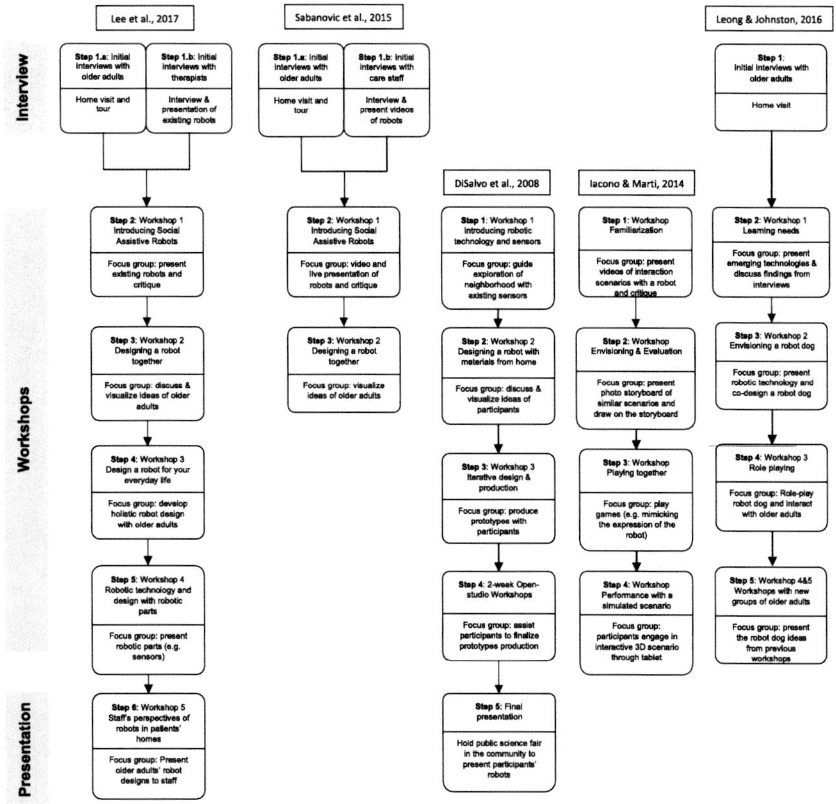

FIGURE 7.2
Examples of HRI participatory design workshop formats with older adults (from: Rogers et al., 2022).

7.2.4 Demonstrating robot capabilities

Most older adults have not had personal experience with robots. Therefore, attention should be given to appropriately demonstrating a robot's abilities when conducting research with older adults and robots. As a robot developer, do you want to assess older adults' perceptions or interactions with robots in an ideal context in which the robot does not fail or make errors or in a realistic context in which the robot might have to make mistakes and learn over time? The answer will depend on both the stage of development and the goal of the research.

In our research, we have had success showing video demonstrations to assess older adults' perceptions about robots. The benefit of using a video is that the researchers have control over how the robot's behavior is presented. For example, ideal robot performance can be demonstrated through editing, omitting errors, and increasing the frame rate. This demonstration would be done not to mislead the participant but rather to assess a participant's attitudes based on the future potential of a robot. Otherwise, the participant may get distracted or too focused on any errors that occur or the slowness of the robot's performance. Alternatively, depending on the researcher's goal, it may be important to highlight realistic aspects of robot performance such as the type of errors it may make or the process required for it to complete a task. Videos can also be an appropriate choice if there is a high risk of safety for in-person interaction.

Much HRI is conducted using robot prototypes, often using a *Wizard of Oz* method. In a *Wizard of Oz* scenario, a researcher is controlling the technology, perhaps unbeknownst to the participant, while the participant conducts a task with the technology. The presence of "Wizard" refers to the robot, and the presence of "Oz" refers to the human. This is a well-established and accepted method for evaluating HRI, particularly when testing a hypothetical system or prototype capability. The researcher can simulate autonomous activities of the robot to test various characteristics of engagement between a robot and a human (e.g., approach, duration, frequency, proximity, physical contact) before programming the robot to interact with the person autonomously in an ideal way. For example, a researcher may want to get user feedback on how a robot optimally approaches someone to assist them to stand from a seated position. Or in the case of understanding human acceptance of a future robot, a researcher may want to understand acceptable and unacceptable characteristics of a bathing robot. These insights inform the development of that robot.

Several variations of the Wizard of Oz experiment method have been outlined (see Figure 7.3). The *Oz of Wizard* simulates the human behavior, often for refining technological functions such as computer vision, machine learning, and artificial intelligence. The *Oz with Wizard* includes human participants but primarily to measure robot performance in the context of a human, not to measure human behavior in response to a robot. This method might be used for measuring robot reliability or accuracy when interacting with or around a human. The *Wizard with Oz* method includes human participants and closely measures their behavior in the context of the robot, but there is no measurement of the robot. While the robot technology is real, aspects of the robot's behavior or the environment might be simulated. This method is often used for measuring human attitudes, comfort, trust, and workload, particularly before deployment. *Wizard and Oz* can be thought of as the ideal method for evaluating HRI and is consistent with immersive participatory design. In this case, the robot and the humans are both real, and they are interacting in a realistic environment; there are no simulated behaviors, and multiple aspects of the interaction can be measured (e.g., human behavior, robot behavior, environmental characteristics). Lastly, in a *Wizard nor Oz* scenario, both human and robot behavior are simulated. As such, this approach would be least ideal, but necessary in certain cases such as when the other methods would pose significant safety risks to the human or damage to the robot.

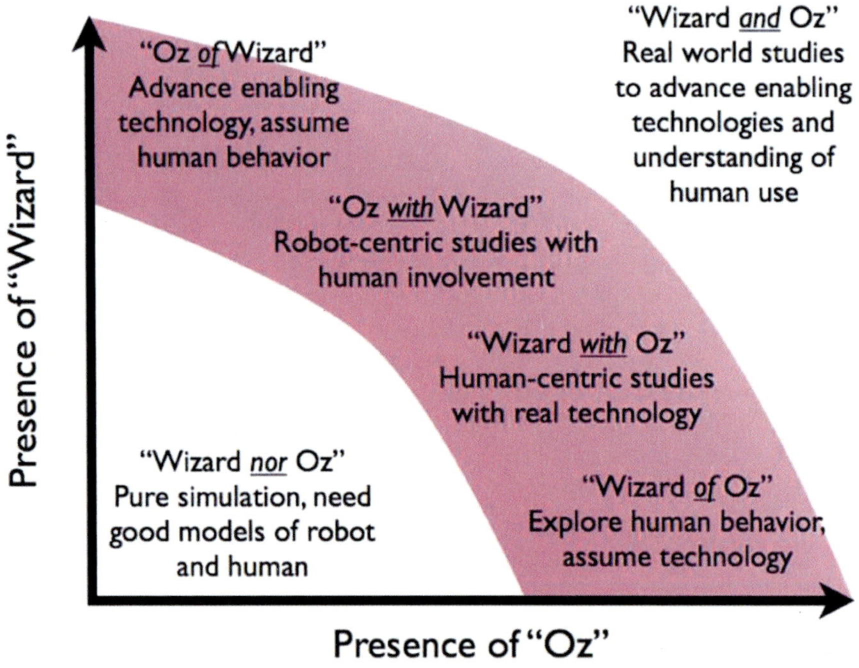

FIGURE 7.3
Wizard/Oz combinations (from: Steinfeld et al., 2009).

7.2.5 Questionnaires, interviews, and focus groups

Research using subjective methods such as questionnaires, interviews, and focus groups can inform understanding of older adults' perceptions, attitudes, acceptance, and beliefs about robots, which can provide rich insights for developers and designers. Questionnaires are useful for collecting data from a large number of people but can be used with smaller samples. Determining sample size for a quantitative research study is complex and is outside of the scope of this chapter. However, for usability studies, 40–60 participants will likely be sufficient for a questionnaire. Traditionally, these studies have been structured with a single set of items and a single-item order or in some cases various counterbalanced orders. However, with online data collection software such as Qualtrics, questions can be more customized to an individual. Questionnaires can be a relatively quick and inexpensive way to collect data when specific questions are known to the researchers as well as the potential response categories.

Interviews can be structured to varying degrees and are more open for personal input from the individuals being interviewed than questionnaires. They can allow researchers to delve deeper into participants' responses with follow-up questions. The number of participants needed for an interview study can range greatly, but typically is around 12–30. A common criterion for determining sufficient sample size in an interview study is data saturation (i.e., the point where collecting additional data does not identify new or unique themes or theoretical insights). Individual interviews can be more appropriate when the topics of interest are designed to bring up personal issues (e.g., needs for personal care or toileting assistance) or when a population of interest is difficult to recruit (e.g., low prevalence in the population). Group interviews, sometimes called focus groups, can be useful for facilitating conversation and idea generation because participants can cue each other. Group interviews typically include four to eight participants, a moderator, and an assistant or notetaker. Several group interviews (two to four) should be conducted to capture the range of relevant issues.

Individual or group interviews may be effective ways to follow up on research findings from a questionnaire study that requires a more in-depth analysis. Interviews can also be useful for designing questionnaires as researchers explore new areas and research questions to help them develop and/or refine meaningful items for a questionnaire. When starting research in a new field or with a new population, it can be helpful to conduct subject matter expert interviews for a high-reward, low-effort way to get a general understanding of relevant issues and terminology.

Using a mixed-methods approach that incorporates both questionnaires and interviews can be optimal for some investigations because the qualitative findings can provide context for and insight into the quantitative results. We conducted a mixed-methods interaction study with the robot, PARO (see Figure 3.2; http://www.parorobots.com), wherein we examined attitudes about, engagement with, and emotions toward PARO for healthy, cognitively intact, independently living older adults. Data were collected in individual sessions with older adult participants. Figure 7.4 depicts the procedural flow wherein qualitative interview data were collected at multiple timepoints (initial reaction, pre-assessment, reassessment reaction, post-assessment), and quantitative questionnaire data were collected as well (pre-assessment, interaction period, post-assessment). The interaction period was video recorded and later coded using qualitative analysis.

These methods can be implemented remotely via online questionnaires and video platforms. As such, a broader range of people may be able to participate, and larger samples can be obtained. However, the technology knowledge needed to participate might lead to a selective sample of tech-savvy participants. Nevertheless, the benefits of more diverse and geographically distributed samples can be informative.

7.2.6 Interaction studies

In an interaction study, a robot interacts with one or more human participants. This may involve data being collected about the robot's behavior and/or the human's behavior or attitudes. The PARO study, introduced above,

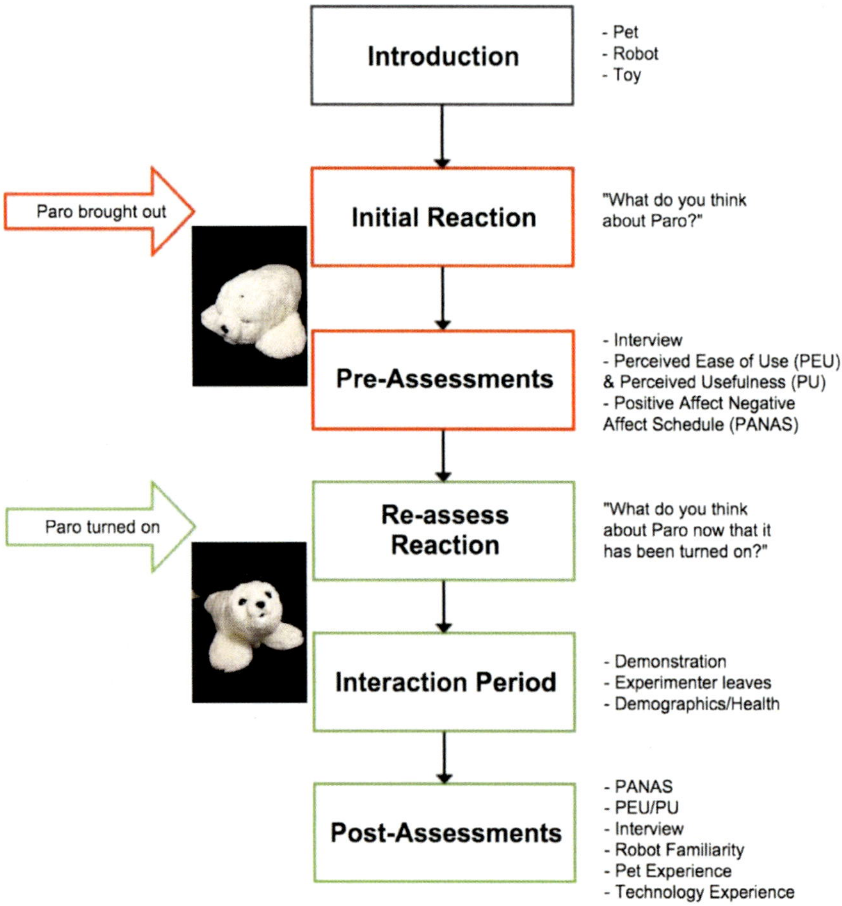

FIGURE 7.4
Procedural flow for mixed-methods investigation of older adults' engagement with PARO robot (from: McGlynn et al., 2017).

was a mixed-methods interaction study. Participants began by completing a set of abilities tests. Next, the experimenter introduced PARO under one of three randomly assigned framing conditions (pet, robot, or toy) and asked for the participant's permission to turn on the video camera and bring PARO out. After PARO (in "off" mode) was placed on the table in front of the participant, they were asked an initial reaction question, "What do you think about the PARO?" The experimenter then administered a short interview and a set of pre-interaction questionnaires. Next, PARO was turned on and the same reaction question was asked again. Following this, the experimenter demonstrated possible interactions with PARO and then asked the participant if they would like to interact with PARO. The experimenter then left the participant in the room alone with PARO for ten minutes, while the participant completed another questionnaire. This short-term exposure period allowed for the potential for interaction (which was video recorded with the participant's permission). After this period, the experimenter returned to the room, PARO was turned off, and the participant completed a post-interaction questionnaire and interview. The video of the interaction period was coded, and a wide range of interactions between the participants and PARO were identified (see Figure 7.5). We found large individual differences in the total number of times older adults actively engaged with PARO, with some engaged several hundred times, and one not engaging with PARO at all. Moreover, those who engaged with PARO more frequently during the interaction period reported more positive affect post-interaction, even when controlling for baseline positive affect. This study demonstrates the value of using qualitative coding of robot interaction in conjunction with questionnaire data.

The benefit of the PARO study being a mixed-methods study was that we collected quantitative data (coded video and questionnaires) to capture

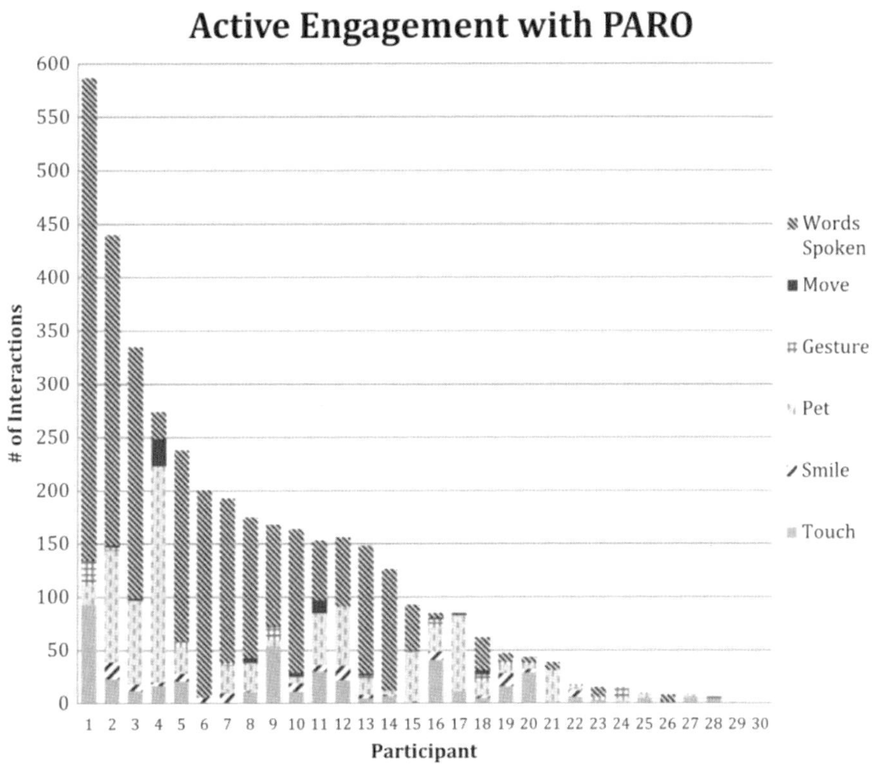

FIGURE 7.5
Total number of interactions for each engagement type listed for each of the participants, ordered from (left) most total interactions to (right) fewest total interactions (from: McGlynn et al., 2017).

the number of interactions and quantify attitudes about the PARO across participants, but we also collected qualitative data from the interviews to provide insight into the attitudes that drove those interactions and attitudes.

Interaction studies can involve multiple participants (depending on the power needed to test a particular hypothesis) or a single case study for rich, detailed data about one individual participant, such as the immersive participatory design case we explore in Chapter 8. The PARO study depicted in Figure 7.5 included 30 participants. Studies focused on usability may only need 10–20 participants, but the participants should be recruited strategically to reflect a range of users (e.g., technology experience). Single case studies can be ideal for unique populations (e.g., rare physical disabilities) or in complex research contexts.

Most interaction studies focused on robots for older adults are short-term engagement studies. Longer-term interaction studies in natural environments are critical to understand how older users engage with robots in their daily lives over time, after any novelty effects have diminished.

7.2.7 Virtual reality and simulation environments

Given the challenges of testing robots in a wide range of situations, there is a trend toward having a digital robot twin that is a virtual representation of the robot – or components of the robot – that is designed to accurately reflect its physical characteristics. This approach enables simulation and comparing different approaches to a robotics challenge. For example, a team at TechSAge (https://techsage.ahs.illinois.edu/d3-soft-robotic-shower-head-sorosh/) is using a robotic simulation platform to provide realistic modeling of a bathroom outfitted with a robotic shower to show older adults and wheelchair users how such a shower might be implemented to gather their input on usability and usefulness. They are able to model the kinematic movements of a human during bathing actions to provide a realistic simulation for user input.

RCareWorld is a simulation platform that has been developed explicitly for evaluating robot caregiving. It includes realistic human modeling, home environments, and assistive robots. As described on their site,

> This simulation is designed using inputs from stakeholders such as expert occupational therapists, care recipients, and caregivers. It models the human avatars with musculoskeletal models and XPBD-based flesh, and builds them with clinical data. It provides a variety of benchmark ADL tasks in realistic settings. It interfaces with various physics engines to model rigid, articulated, and deformable objects. It provides the capability to plan, control, and learn human and robot control policies by interfacing with state-of-the-art external planning and learning libraries.
>
> *(https://emprise.cs.cornell.edu/rcareworld/)*

These approaches allow for evaluation of a range of scenarios to illustrate different consequences of implementing robotics with older users. As discussed in Chapter 6, consideration of a various situations can help inform understanding of potential ethical issues.

7.3 Measures

We will discuss a variety of questionnaires to assess HRI issues including acceptance, trust, negative attitudes, assistance preferences, appearance, familiarity and use, usability, and general HRI. Some of these measures are described in a technical report (see Rogers & Mitzner, 2015) that included details about the questionnaire development, instructions for administration and scoring, as well as details on modifications and revisions. Others are included in the recommended readings at the end of the chapter. When selecting a measure, consider both the validity (i.e., its accuracy or how well it measures what it is supposed to measure) and the reliability (i.e., its consistency or how well it controls random error to repeatedly reproduce the same results).

7.3.1 Acceptance

The purpose of the Robot Opinions Questionnaire is to assess attitudinal robot acceptance, specifically regarding perceptions of usefulness and ease of use. This questionnaire can be administered before or after interacting with a robot, or both before and after to assess changes in pre-post preferences (Smarr et al., 2014). The questionnaire was based on standard technology acceptance scales developed to measure the perceptions of usefulness and ease of use (Davis, 1989). The questionnaire consists of 12 opinion statements about robots: 6 related to usefulness and 6 related to ease of use. Each statement is presented with a seven-point scale that corresponds to levels of agreement with the statement: 1 = extremely unlikely; 2 = quite unlikely; 3 = slightly unlikely; 4 = neither likely nor unlikely; 5 = slightly likely; 6 = quite likely; 7 = extremely likely. Given that most people will not have robot experience, the instructions state to "Imagine that you have the opportunity to use or operate a robot. Please place an X in the response box that best represents your general opinion (we understand that there may be exceptions)." This questionnaire is easily modifiable to specific populations. For example, we measured robot acceptance of professional caregivers of older adults, modifying the usefulness items to reflect the usefulness of a robot for caregiving tasks (e.g., "Using a robot would make my daily life easier" was changed to "Using a robot would make caregiving tasks easier."). This questionnaire can also be modified to add additional dimensions of technology acceptance including enjoyment, subjective norm, and trust.

7.3.2 Trust

Trust is a complex construct that includes both the capability and reliability of the robot to be trusted and the willingness of the user to be vulnerable. Trust can also be affected by the task and the environment. Hence, measures designed to assess trust between humans and robots can vary widely and should be selected based on the specific research question at hand. Many trust measures originated in the automation literature. Trust in automation has been measured with behavioral indices such as compliance, agreement rate, decision time, reliance, and response time, as well as physiological measures such as electrodermal activity, eye gazing, heart rate change and variability, and neural measures. Nevertheless, self-report is the most frequently reported method for measuring trust in automation as well as trust in HRI (see Table 7.1 for a list of self-report measures of trust). Note that the Multi-Dimensional Measure of Trust (MDMT) and the Trust Perception Scale for Human–Robot Interaction were designed specifically to capture trust in robots. Trust is frequently measured via subscales of technology acceptance questionnaires, such as the Robot Opinions Questionnaire described earlier.

7.3.3 Negative attitudes

The Negative Attitude toward Robots Scale is a questionnaire designed to measure the attitudes and emotions of people about interacting with robots that may be barriers to interaction (Nomura et al., 2006). The scale is composed of three subscales: negative attitudes toward situations of interaction with robots, negative attitudes toward the social influence of robots, and negative attitudes toward emotions in interaction with robots. For each of the 17 items, participants are presented with a five-point scale to indicate agreement, from 1 = I strongly disagree to 5 = I strongly agree.

7.3.4 Assistance preferences

The purpose of the Assistance Preference Checklist is to assess how preferences for human assistance versus robot assistance vary as a function of task, and perhaps change over time. It can be administered before or after interacting with a robot, or both before and after to assess changes in pre-post preferences. One version of task checklist consists of 58 Likert scale items, all beginning with the phrase: "If I needed assistance, I would prefer help from…" (Smarr et al., 2014). This phrase is followed by a list of tasks for which a user may need assistance, such as bathing or doing laundry, with response options for assistance preference: 1 = only a human; 2 = prefer a human; 3 = no preference; 4 = prefer a robot; 5 = only a robot. See Figure 7.6 for the

TABLE 7.1

Self-report measures of trust

Measure	Original Source	Relevant Construct
Checklist for Trust	Jian et al. (2000)	Factors of perceived trustworthiness; trust
Complacency Potential Rating Scale	Singh et al. (1993)	Trustor's propensity
Dynamic Reporting of Trust	Desai (2012)	Trust
Human-Computer Trust (HCT) Questionnaire	Madsen and Gregor (2000)	Factors of perceived trustworthiness; trust
Individual Differences in Trust in Automation	Varied	Trustor's propensity
Integrated Model of Trust	Muir and Moray (1996)	Trust
Measures of Trust and Trustworthiness	Mayer and Davis (1999)	Factors of perceived trustworthiness; trust (Propensity and outcomes not frequently used)
MDMT	Malle and Ullman (2021)	Factors of perceived trustworthiness; trust
Self-Reports of Automation Qualities (Reliability, Accuracy)	None	Factors of perceived trustworthiness
Trust and Self-Confidence Scale	Lee and Moray (1994)	Trust
Trust in Automated Systems Test (TOAST)	Wojton et al. (2020)	Factors of perceived trustworthiness
Trust in Automation Scale	Körber et al. (2015)	Factors of perceived trustworthiness; trust
Trust Perception Scale for Human–Robot Interaction (HRI)	Schaefer (2016)	Factors of perceived trustworthiness; trust
Trust Scale (1)	Lee and Moray (1992)	Trust
Trust Scale (2)	Merritt (2011)	Factors of perceived trustworthiness; trust

Source: Adapted from: Kohn et al. (2021) and relevant construct Mayer and Davis (1999).

instructions and example items. Note that it is important to provide a context such as "imagine you need assistance" when assessing older users' attitudes about robotic support. In our work, we have found that by only asking older adults if they would like assistance from a robot, they might say "no" and explain that they do not need any assistance at all.

In another version of the questionnaire, we modified the task checklist to reflect the tasks that are frequently performed by healthcare providers caring for older adults. The healthcare providers study version categorized tasks into the following sections: activities of daily living (nine questions), instrumental activities of daily living (five questions), medical tasks (seven

Assistance Preference Checklist

We are interested in learning about older adults' preferences for assistance in performing daily living tasks. In particular, we are looking for opinions about human assistance and robot assistance. When completing this questionnaire, please imagine you need assistance in everyday life with various tasks.

For each of the following tasks, please provide your opinion about your:

- Preference for human assistance
- No preference
- Preference for robot assistance

Assume that the robot could perform the task to the level of a human. Please circle the most appropriate response for your general preference (we understand that there may be exceptions).

On the last page, there is space for you to provide additional comments about your preferences for having robot and human assistance.

If I needed assistance with...	If I needed assistance, I would prefer help from...				
	Only a human$_1$	Prefer a human$_2$	No Preference	Prefer a robot$_4$	Only a robot$_5$
a. Bathing	1	2	3	4	5
b. Being entertained (e.g., playing games, dancing)	1	2	3	4	5
c. Being reminded of appointments	1	2	3	4	5
d. Being reminded of daily activities	1	2	3	4	5
e. Being reminded to take medicine	1	2	3	4	5
f. Brushing teeth	1	2	3	4	5
g. Calling doctors/911	1	2	3	4	5

FIGURE 7.6
Assistance Preference Checklist instructions and example items (from: Smarr et al., 2014).

questions), device use (14 questions), and administrative and communication tasks (four questions; Mitzner et al., 2018). The results from using both versions are discussed in Chapter 2 (see Figure 2.5).

7.3.5 Appearance preferences

Attitudes about robot appearance have been explored using questionnaires, such as how humanlike, mechanical, likable, threatening, submissive, or unfamiliar they are perceived. For example, there is an online estimation tool researchers can use to predict how humanlike a new robot will be perceived given the presence of various features (http://www.abotdatabase.info; Phillips et al., 2018). The tool is based on a database called ABOT (Anthropomorphic roBOT), which is a collection of 250 images of real-world anthropomorphic robots.

Robot appearance influences a person's response to robots, as evidenced by the Robotic Social Attributes Scale (RoSAS; Stroessner & Benitez, 2019). For example, artificial robot faces that were feminine (versus masculine) and humanlike (versus machinelike) were judged as warmer and produced higher levels of comfort, which were associated with more positive evaluations and greater desire for engagement.

7.3.6 Familiarity and use experience

The purpose of the Robot Familiarity and Use Questionnaire is to assess the extent of familiarity and use experience one has with different types of robots. The questionnaire included 13 robot categories: autonomous car, domestic or home robot, entertainment or toy robot, manufacturing robot, military robot, Personal Robot 2 (PR2; discussed in Chapter 2), remote presence robot, research robot, robot lawn mower, space exploration robot, robot security guard, surgical robot, and unmanned aerial vehicle. Participants are presented with a five-point scale to indicate their familiarity with each of these categories of robots: 0 = not sure what this is; 1 = never heard about, seen, or used this robot; 2 = only heard about or seen this robot; 3 = used or operated this robot only occasionally; 4 = used or operated this robot frequently (Smarr et al., 2014). Given the growing numbers of robots being developed, the robot examples should be evaluated and modified based on the current market availability.

7.3.7 Usability

In one scoping review, seven questionnaires were identified for evaluating the usability of robots (Moulaei et al., 2024). Two – The System Usability Scale and the User Experience Questionnaire – were the most frequently administered questionnaires. The System Usability Scale is a questionnaire designed to measure perceived usability of a system or product. It consists of ten items that focus on different dimensions of usability including ease of use, efficiency, satisfaction, and learnability. Participants are presented with a five-point scale with higher scores indicating higher usability. Total scores are then averaged and scaled to get a final score. Typical benchmarks are 68 (average usability) and 80 (above average usability).

The User Experience Questionnaire was designed to measure six user experience and usability-related factors: attractiveness, perspicuity, efficiency, dependability, stimulation, and novelty (Laugwitz et al., 2008). It consists of 26 items that measure both traditional usability factors and user experience factors.

In our research, we have used the NASA Task Load Index, or TLX (Hart, 2006) as a measure of usability. The NASA TLX assesses usability across six dimensions (mental demand, physical demand, temporal demand, effort, performance, frustration level) to determine an overall workload rating. Participants are asked to rate their score on an interval scale ranging from low (1) to high

(20). Lastly, we have included usability items (e.g., "I would find a robot easy to use") in the Robot Opinions Questionnaire in some of our studies.

7.3.8 General HRI perceptions

Some general HRI perception measures have been developed, the most common of which is the Godspeed Questionnaire (Bartneck et al., 2009), which measures five concepts in HRI: (1) anthropomorphism (the attribution of human features and behaviors to a robots); (2) animacy (that attribution of life to the robot); (3) likeability (the attribution of friendliness to the robot); (4) perceived intelligence (the attribution of intellectual competence to the robot); and (5) perceived safety (how anxious the perceiver feels in response to the robot). Participants indicate their responses to items on scales anchored by two opposing words (e.g., artificial and lifelike).

The Robot Social Attributes Scale is another general HRI measure designed to assess fundamental social reactions to robots (Carpinella et al., 2017). It was built upon the Godspeed Questionnaire but designed to be a more psychometrically valid scale of robot social perception. It includes 18 items to characterize judgments of robots, reflecting the dimensions of warmth, competence, and discomfort. Participants respond using a nine-point scale from 1 = definitely not associated to 9 = definitely associated.

7.4 Guidelines for design methods and assessment measures

- Consider the range of stakeholders that should be represented in your assessments.
- Design evaluation materials to be accessible to people with different abilities and disabilities.
- Use personas to gain insights about older adults' specific needs, goals, preferences, and everyday activities and behaviors.
- Involve older adults in the design process to the degree possible.
- Carefully select a method for demonstrating a robot's capabilities; consider whether it should show ideal behavior or realistic behavior.
- Use questionnaires to collect data when specific questions and potential response categories are known.
- Use interviews to collect rich details and contextual understanding of attitudes and behaviors.
- Conduct interviews with subject matter experts when starting research in a new field or with a new population.
- When designing interaction studies, consider whether to control the context or environment of the HRI and whether to control or measure the behavior of the robot.

- Consider timing of HRI measures: whether measures should be administered one time or both pre- and post-interaction, if assessing possible changes.

Recommended readings and links

Readings

Bartneck, C., Croft, E., Kulic, D., & Zoghbi, S. (2009). Measurement instruments for the anthropomorphism, animacy, likeability, perceived intelligence, and perceived safety of robots. *International Journal of Social Robotics*, 1(1) 71–81. https://doi.org/10.1007/s12369-008-0001-3

Bayles, M. A., Mitzner, T. L., & Rogers, W. A. (2021). *TechSAge Tool: Conducting research with older adults aging with sensory and mobility disabilities*. Rehabilitation Engineering Research Center on Technologies to Support Aging-in-Place for People with Long-Term Disabilities. https://techsage.gatech.edu/sites/default/files/2022-01/TechSAge%20Tool_ResearchGuide.pdf

Brooke, J. (1996). SUS—A quick and dirty usability scale. *Usability Evaluation in Industry, 189*, 4–7. https://doi.org/10.1201/9781498710411-35

Carpinella, C. M., Wyman, A. B., Perez, M. A., & Stroessner, S. J. (2017). The robotic social attributes scale (RoSAS): Development and validation. *Proceedings of the 2017 ACM/IEEE International Conference on Human-Robot Interaction*, Vienna, Austria, pp. 254–262

Davis, F. D. (1989). Perceived usefulness, perceived ease of use, and user acceptance of information technology. *MIS Quarterly, 13*(3), 319–340. https://doi.org/10.2307/249008

Hart, S. G. (2006). NASA-task load index (NASA-TLX): 20 Years later. *Proceedings of the Human Factors and Ergonomic Society Annual Meeting, 50*, 904–908.

Kohn, S. C., de Visser, E. J., Wiese, E., Lee, Y. C., & Shaw, T. H. (2021). Measurement of trust in automation: A narrative review and reference guide. *Frontiers in Psychology, 12*, 604977. https://doi.org/10.3389/fpsyg.2021.604977

Laugwitz, B., Held, T., & Schrepp, M. (2008). USAB 2008, LNCS 5298. In *Construction and evaluation of a user experience questionnaire*. Symposium of the Austrian HCI and Usability Engineering Group (pp. 63–76).

McGlynn, S. A., Kemple, S., Mitzner, T. L., King, C. A., & Rogers, W. A. (2017). Understanding the potential of PARO for healthy older adults. *International Journal of Human-Computer Studies, 100*, 33–47. https://doi.org/10.1016/j.ijhcs.2016.12.004

Mitzner, T. L., Tiberio, L., Kemp, C. C., & Rogers, W. A. (2018). Understanding healthcare providers' perceptions of a personal assistant robot. *Gerontechnology, 17*(1), 48–55. https://doi.org/10.4017/gt.2018.17.1.005.00

Moulaei, K., Moulaei, R., & Bahaadinbeigy, K. (2024). The most used questionnaires for evaluating the usability of robots and smart wearables: A scoping review. *Digital Health, 10*, 20552076241237384. https://doi.org/10.1177/20552076241237384

Nomura, T., Suzuki, T., Kanda, T., & Kato, K. (2006). Measurement of negative attitudes toward robots. *Interaction Studies, 7*, 437–454.

Olatunji, S. A., Nguyen, V., Cakmak, M., Edsinger, A., Kemp, C. C., Rogers, W. A., & Mahajan, H. P. (2024). Immersive participatory design of assistive robots to support older adults. *Ergonomics, 67*(6), 717–731. https://doi.org/10.1080/00140139.2024.2312529

Rogers, W. A., Kadylak, T., & Bayles, M. A. (2022). Maximizing the benefits of participatory design for human-robot interaction research with older adults. *Human Factors, 64*(3), 441–450. https://doi.org/10.1177/00187208211037465

Rogers, W. A., & Mitzner, T. L. (2015). *Survey instruments for robotics research in the Human Factors and Aging Laboratory (HFA-TR-1501)*. Atlanta: Georgia Institute of Technology, School of Psychology, Human Factors and Aging Laboratory.

Smarr, C. A., Mitzner, T. L., Beer, J. M., Prakash, A., Chen, T. L., Kemp, C. C., & Rogers, W. A. (2014). Domestic robots for older adults: Attitudes, preferences, and potential. *International Journal of Social Robotics, 6*(2), 229–247.

Stroessner, S. J., & Benitez, J. (2019). The social perception of humanoid and non-humanoid robots: Effects of gendered and machinelike features. *International Journal of Social Robotics, 11*(2), 305–315. https://doi.org/10.1007/s12369-018-0502-7

TechSAge. (2017). *TechSAge Tool: Personas for designing for individuals aging with mobility impairment*. Rehabilitation Engineering Research Center on Technologies to Support Aging-in-Place for People with Long-Term Disabilities. https://techsage.gatech.edu/sites/default/files/2021-01/Design%20Personas%20TS%20Tool_0.pdf

Vargas, C., Whelan, J., Brimblecombe, J., & Allender, S. (2022). Co-creation, co-design and co-production for public health: A perspective on definitions and distinctions. *Public Health Research and Practice,* 32(2), e3222211. https://doi.org/10.17061/phrp3222211

Links

Design of a Soft Robotic Shower Head (SoRoSH):
https://techsage.ahs.illinois.edu/d3-soft-robotic-shower-head-sorosh/

Etiquette: Interacting with people with disabilities:
https://www.respectability.org/inclusion-toolkits/etiquette-interacting-with-people-with-disabilities/

Guide to interacting with disabilities:
https://www.dhs.state.il.us/OneNetLibrary/27897/documents/Brochures/4151.pdf

Predictor to forecast the extent to which a robot will be perceived as humanlike:
https://www.abotdatabase.info/predictor

Putting a face on a robot:
https://phys.org/news/2013-10-robot.html

RCareWorld: A human-centric simulation world for caregiving robots:
https://emprise.cs.cornell.edu/rcareworld/

TechSAge Tool: Personas for designing for individuals aging with mobility impairment:
https://techsage.gatech.edu/sites/default/files/2021-01/Design%20Personas%20TS%20Tool_0.pdf

8

Applying the HRI framework: the Evans story

8.1 Overview of applications

The goal for this chapter is to provide an application case study that illustrates how the dimensions of the human–robot interaction (HRI) framework can be used to guide robot design. We will illustrate how the characteristics of the human(s), the robot, the interaction, and the environmental context influenced the design process. We will describe the methods and measures used to evaluate the robot in this context in terms of acceptance and effectiveness. We will discuss ethical considerations and provide lessons learned. This case study illustrates the complexities of designing a robot to be used in a home setting by a family with unique needs and highlights the benefits of using immersive participatory design.

8.2 The Evans family and the Stretch robot: a case study

Henry and Jane Evans are willing to share their story because they believe in the potential of robots to support the independence and autonomy of people living with physical support needs. They will be the first to say that robots have changed their lives, and recently one robot, in particular. The Stretch® robot was developed by Hello Robot, co-founded by Dr. Aaron Edsinger and Dr. Charlie Kemp in 2017, with the goal of advancing the design of robots that have impact on people's lives. This chapter presents a case study of the Evans family and their use and evaluation of the Stretch robot. (*Conflict of interest notes*: Wendy Rogers is an advisor to Hello Robot, Inc., and co-investigator on grants with them [https://hello-robot.com/about]. However, she does not have any financial interest in the company. Also note that Dr. Kemp wrote the Foreword for this book.)

DOI: 10.1201/9781032656649-8

8.2.1 Introducing Henry and Jane Evans

Henry and Jane Evans were married in 1987 (see Figure 8.1). They built a life together and had four children. They had recently built their dream home in the hills of Los Altos, outside of San Francisco, when in 2002, at 40 years old, Henry experienced a brain stem dissection (likely there since birth) that resulted in severe loss of function. After years of physical therapy, he can sit up for extended periods in his bed or wheelchair and has limited use of one thumb, but he is mute with quadriplegia. At the time of Henry's health event, Jane was raising their children who were aged 6, 8, 12, and 13. Together the family made the decision to set up their home in such a way that Henry could remain there – Jane is his primary caregiver with support from professional caregivers.

In 2010, Henry saw a news report on CNN about a personal robot that was developed by Willow Garage called the Personal Robot 2 (PR2). A team at the Georgia Institute of Technology led by Professors Charlie Kemp and Wendy Rogers was exploring the potential of the PR2 to support people in their homes. Henry tracked down the CEO of Willow Garage, Steve Cousins, who connected him to Charlie Kemp, and a partnership was born. Henry and Jane have been engaged in robotics research since then, establishing the Robots for Humanity initiative (https://r4h.org/). For more about their story, see "This Robot Could Be the Key to Empowering People with Disabilities" (https://spectrum.ieee.org/stretch-assistive-robot).

As discussed in Chapter 2, the HRI stakeholders' capabilities and limitations need to be considered during the design of the robot. Not all the human characteristics in the framework will be relevant to every case. Here we will focus on Henry as a robot user and care recipient; Jane as a robot user and care provider; and on them both as a team (referred to collectively as "Henry

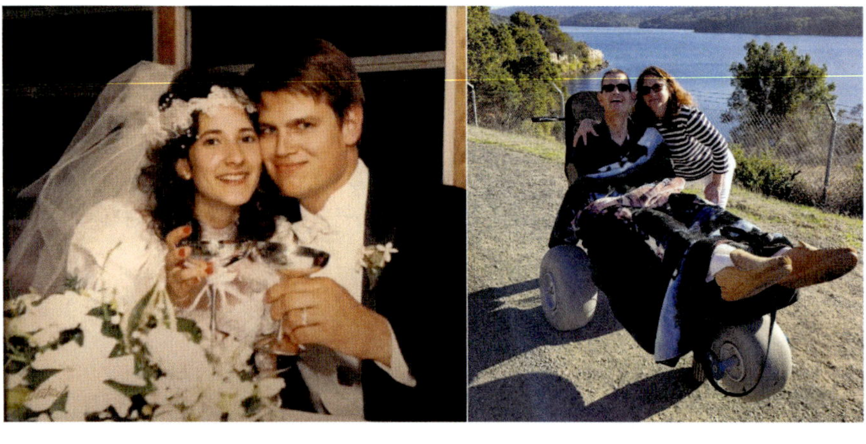

FIGURE 8.1
Meet Henry and Jane Evans.

and Jane"). They work together daily to perform tasks that contribute to their quality of life, which includes activities of daily living (ADLs), instrumental ADLs (IADLs), and enhanced ADLs (EADLs), as described in Chapter 4.

8.2.1.1 Henry

Henry is a 63-year-old male with a master's degree in business. His cognitive and perceptual abilities are completely intact. His motor abilities are severely limited. He cannot walk or talk but has some use of one thumb that he uses to control a joystick on the computer. He uses a head tracker and click-switch to control computer interfaces or communicates with a manual letter board. He has a high level of user experience with technology including robots – he regularly uses telepresence robots and has been engaged in robotics research for over a decade.

8.2.1.2 Jane

Jane is a 61-year-old female with a college education. She is generally healthy with intact cognitive, perceptual, and motor abilities. She is managing a chronic health condition. She is relatively tech-savvy and experienced with robots (although perhaps less than Henry). She has deep familiarity with the domain of caregiving tasks.

8.2.1.3 Henry and Jane

With respect to psychosocial characteristics, both Henry and Jane are positive people with excellent senses of humor. As might be imagined for people in their situation, they deal with the demands of daily caregiving needs, and their moods may vary depending on the circumstances of the day. They have high self-efficacy with respect to confidence in working with robots. They have very clear preferences that influence their ideas for how the robot should perform and the capabilities it should have. Their experiences with robots in general, and Stretch in particular, influence their trust in the Stretch robot to perform different tasks.

8.2.2 Introducing Stretch the robot

Stretch is a mobile manipulator robot whose development has involved several iterations; here, we focus on Stretch 3, depicted in Figure 8.2. Using Chapter 3 as a guide, we review the features of the Stretch robot that are most relevant to the interactions that Henry and Jane will have with it.

Stretch was designed to support tasks in domestic environments. It is relatively lightweight (~51 lbs) with a small footprint to maneuver through small spaces. It is a machinelike robot with a telescoping arm that enables it to stretch (hence the name) to pick items up from the floor or on a counter.

Stretch can hold different tools, be outfitted with different end effectors, and can hold a tablet to display information. Stretch has a mobile base and can learn the layout of different environments. In terms of technical specifications, Stretch is open source, has calibrated a unified robotics description format, a gripper, cameras that provide depth and color information, a navigation laser, a microphone array, and an integrated computer (detailed specifications are available here: https://hello-robot.com/stretch-3-product).

With respect to the socialness characteristics of Stretch, they are minimal. Stretch does not display affect or a personality and is generally rated low on the sociability scale. In the Kadylak et al. (2023) study discussed in Chapter 3 (see Figure 3.7), Stretch was rated a 3.29 on a scale of 1 (low sociability) to 7 (high sociability). It would not be considered empathic, does not yet engage in dialogue, and is not proactive in its interactions. However, as additional functions such as voice interaction and sound effects are added to Stretch, these ratings will likely change.

With respect to autonomy, Stretch has multiple modes. It can be fully teleoperated with a game controller or with an onscreen interface (which enables remote operation). Stretch is capable of simple autonomous, user-initiated tasks such as picking up an object or wiping a surface. Stretch can be semi-autonomous for specific tasks; for example, it could autonomously navigate to a specific location and then be controlled by the human to perform a task such as feeding a person.

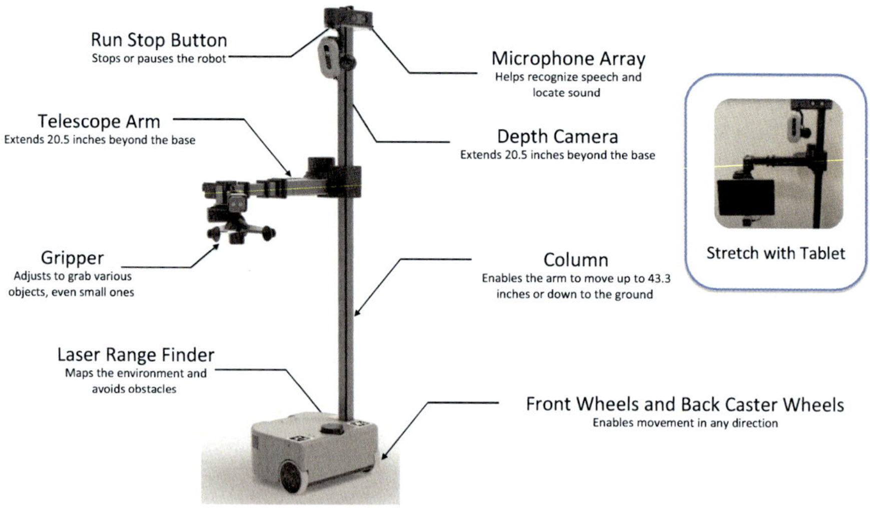

FIGURE 8.2
Meet Stretch the robot (https://hello-robot.com/stretch-3-product). Inset shows Stretch with a tablet computer on the arm.

8.2.3 Interaction

The interaction section of our HRI framework described in Chapter 4 (see Figure 4.1) illustrated the range of things that need to be considered for a robot to be placed in the Evans home to support their caregiving needs.

- *Task characteristics*: The types of tasks that Henry and Jane need support for cover the range of ADLs (e.g., feeding, hygiene), IADLs (e.g., health management, housekeeping), and EADLs (e.g., playing games, social engagement). These tasks impose a variety of constraints, and many require use of a device or tool. Certain tasks have high criticality as they may impact the level of Henry's care.
- *Roles*: In this use case, Henry and Jane may serve all roles (operator, teammate, supervisor, bystander), depending on the task. For example, Henry might operate the robot to scratch an itch; he and Stretch might work together to put laundry in a basket; he may supervise Stretch autonomously navigating to the laundry room; and Jane may be nearby as a bystander. Similarly, Jane might teleoperate Stretch from the kitchen to check on Henry, work together with Stretch to grab something he dropped, or supervise the autonomous delivery of an item to his bed with Henry as the bystander.
- *Engagement*: Given the goals of supporting Henry and Jane in their everyday activities, they will be interacting closely with Stretch, necessitating consideration of all the components, namely, approach, duration, frequency, proximity, and physical contact.
- *Workload*: Considerations of cognitive, physical, and temporal workload are important for both Henry and Jane. The incorporation of Stretch into their lives should not place undue burden on either of them. Nevertheless, using Stretch will require cognitive effort to learn to use it and to control it, physical effort to interact with it, and temporal effort for some tasks that are time sensitive. From Henry's perspective, the use of Stretch should not result in fatigue that interferes with his functional abilities. From Jane's perspective, Stretch should make her tasks easier, and not add caregiver burden.

Considering these interaction components of the HRI framework has provided guidance for the design of Stretch. For instance, there may be multiple ways to perform a task – what is the best approach given the user and the potential for undue workload? If a device needs to be used, how might it be reconfigured to make it easier for Stretch to hold it and for Henry to use it to achieve his goal?

In addition, interaction considerations provided insights regarding the nature of the measures we should include during the evaluations of Stretch. What are the users' feelings about the approach, proximity, and physical contact, and how does that influence their trust in Stretch? How does their role (e.g., operator vs. teammate) influence their workload?

8.2.4 Environments

The environments for this case study include all aspects discussed in Chapter 5 and influenced the design considerations and use evaluations. They are discussed briefly here.

- The *Built Environment* was the Evans home. The main living area is all on one floor, so stairs were not a barrier. The thresholds from room to room were generally low, although some of them did create challenges for moving between rooms. The hallway was relatively narrow but, because it had to accommodate a wheelchair, it could also easily accommodate Stretch. There was, of course, furniture to move around and a variety of rooms to be negotiated. Henry's bedroom, in particular, had limited space for movement given the size of the hospital bed and the healthcare equipment in the room. There were ramps from the indoor spaces to the outdoor spaces, some of which were rather steep. With these considerations in mind, it was critical to ensure that Stretch could easily navigate and did not topple.
- The *Social Environment* included Henry and Jane as well as professional caregivers who would be interacting with the robot. In addition, in the role of bystanders to the HRIs would be family members and friends who were frequent visitors to the home.
- The *Technology Environment* comprised things that might be found in anyone's home such as Henry's and Jane's computers, smartphones, and smart home technologies (e.g., lights, security, digital home assistants). Unique to their home is healthcare equipment such as the percussion vest, hospital bed, various lifts, and a shower chair.
- The *Natural Environment* is relevant to this case study as Henry likes to be outdoors, and ideally Stretch would be there with him to provide support. Their outdoor environment has grass, gravel, pavement, and dirt paths, and is partly hilly.

8.2.5 Introducing the research and development team

Much like it takes a village to raise a child, it takes a team to design, develop, test, and implement a robot in a home environment. Our team has evolved over the years, but our current team is depicted in Figure 8.3. This research is funded by the National Institutes of Health (National Institute on Aging) through a Phase II Small Business Innovation Research (SBIR) Grant entitled "Stretching Their Reach: Robotic Support for Older Individuals with Mild Cognitive Impairment, Early Alzheimer's Dementia, and Mobility

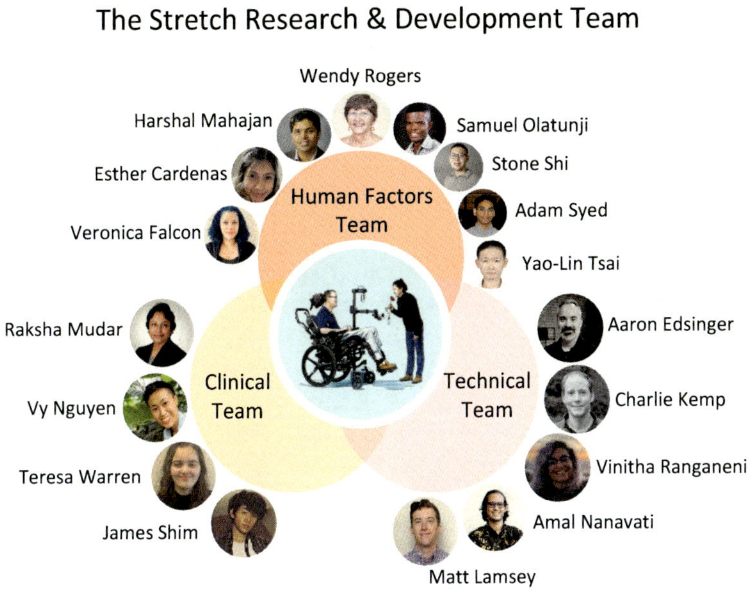

FIGURE 8.3
Meet the research and development team.

Impairments" (R44AG072982), that built on a successful Phase I SBIR grant (R43AG072982). The focus of the case study presented here is for individuals with mobility impairments and their care team. Our work engaging older adults with cognitive impairments is ongoing.

As is clear, Henry and Jane are at the core of the team. Surrounding them are the human factors team, the technical team, and the clinical team. This project represents team science – individuals from different disciplines working together to address a scientific challenge with a shared goal. Such collaborations are not easy given the varied backgrounds, working styles, terminology, disciplinary cultures, personalities, and regional distances. Coordination and communication are core values of the team working to tackle a complex societal issue – namely, providing robotic support to enhance quality of life.

8.2.6 Methods of evaluation and results

We conducted in-home assessments with iterative designs of Stretch in the Evans home for three consecutive summers. Herein we provide an amalgamation of these efforts to illustrate our approach and what we have learned. See the recommended readings for more details about these activities. Our team coined the term "immersive participatory design" to represent our approach to working with the Evans to evaluate Stretch in their home (see Chapter 7 for more details). We drew our measures from occupational therapy, human factors, and HRI. The objective was to have measures that would be specific to Henry and Jane's needs and that would be meaningful in the context of standard metrics reported in the literature.

8.2.6.1 Goals

We used the *Canadian Occupational Performance Measure* (COPM; Law et al., 2019) to assess areas where Stretch could support Henry and Jane and to evaluate their perceptions of using Stretch. The COPM is utilized by occupational therapists to evaluate individual occupational problems and encompasses three areas: self-care, productivity, and leisure activities, which map generally on to ADLs, IADLs, and EADLs, respectively. The COPM includes two ratings scaled from 1 to 10. Performance is how the participants would rate the way they did the activity (1 = not able to do it all to 10 = able to do it extremely well), and satisfaction is how satisfied they were with the way they did the activity (1 = not satisfied at all to 10 = extremely satisfied).

We used the COPM to identify the problems that were important to Henry and Jane and to select tasks that Stretch could assist with that would be meaningful to each of them. We identified important tasks each for Henry (e.g., retrieving snacks from the kitchen for self-feeding, maintaining comfort, social participation with friends and granddaughter) and for Jane (e.g., engaging in exercise, reminders to take blood pressure and learn Spanish, remote caregiving for Henry).

In some cases, we needed to adapt tools such as building up the handle of a hairbrush and spoon to enhance Stretch's ability to grip the materials and to promote the robot user's achievement toward their goals. One overarching goal was Henry's Caregiver Principle:

> No matter how much assistance a device provides to a patient, it will not be used regularly unless it also takes no time to set up or to use by the caregiver, and unless it makes the caregiver's life, overall, a lot easier.

Henry did not want the use of a robot (or any other technology in the home) to impose any burden on Jane (Figure 8.4).

Henry and Jane performed each task without using Stretch and then again using Stretch. Using the COPM scales, we collected pre- and post-use evaluations. Henry's performance on his five tasks increased from 1.2 to 8.2 and his satisfaction from 1.4 to 8.6. Henry used Stretch's gripper for object manipulation such as grasping a spoon for self-feeding or a ball to play with his granddaughters, which both improved his performance of the tasks and increased his level of satisfaction. Henry's improved play and bonding with his granddaughter was a significant achievement. He expressed that when his granddaughter was

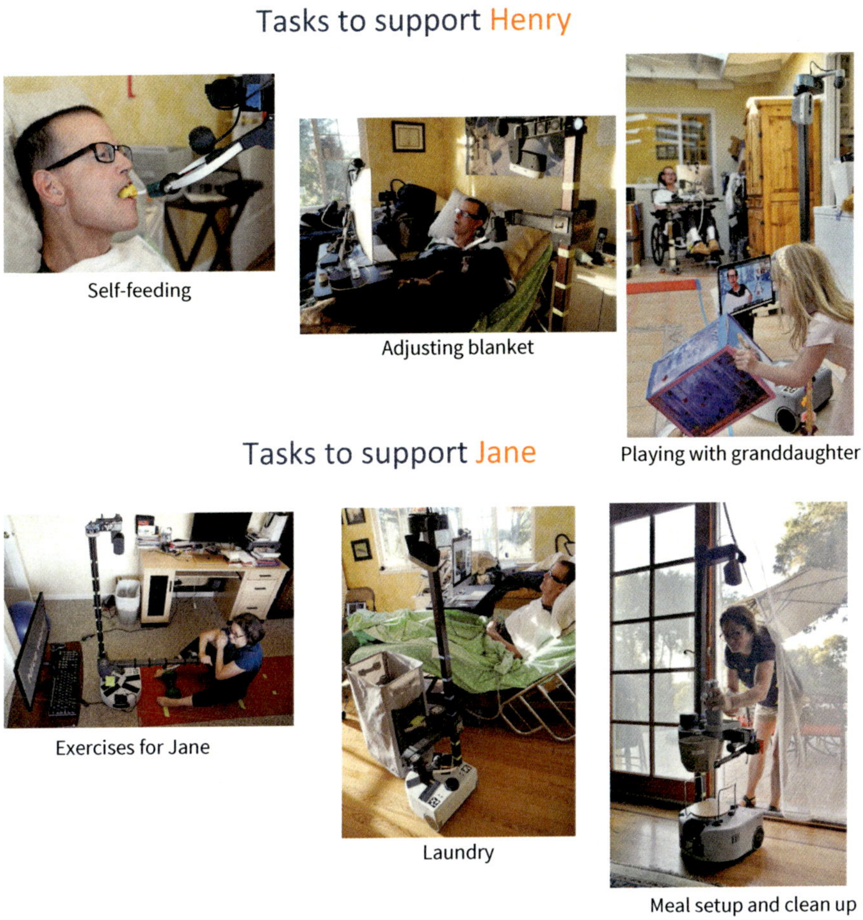

FIGURE 8.4
Sample tasks explored for Henry (top) and Jane (bottom).

> playing games, she immediately started talking directly to me and including me in her games. She has never done that before. It was cool – if we can reproduce that effect with other kids with Stretch, it's a pretty big deal.

For Jane, her performance improved from 5 to 9 and her satisfaction from 4 to 10. For remote caregiving, Jane used autonomous navigation on the user interface to locate Henry's room and instruct a professional caregiver how to put on Henry's bedtime booties using a video call facilitated by Stretch's tablet. Scheduled reminders for blood pressure checks and water intake improved Jane's adherence to this health routine. Jane stated,

> Other things are in my head besides drinking [water], and if I have a reminder with the robot presenting me water on a tray, that's all I need; otherwise, I won't tell myself to hydrate, unless it gets really bad.

These iterative, participatory design sessions demonstrated significant improvements in task performance and satisfaction and provided guidance for design iterations.

With respect to self-feeding, we used an adaptive silicone spoon and plate for Henry to self-feed thick-pureed foods using Stretch. He reported, "I can see myself doing this every evening after dinner for dessert." Jane said,

> Knowing that he had control of Stretch and seeing the silicone spoon he was using, made me feel safe to leave him alone. While he was eating, I was washing dishes. I wouldn't get a chance to do that until later if I was feeding him.

It was critical to choose tools that were safe for Stretch-user interactions and to ensure the environment was clear of safety hazards, such as loose cords or liquids. Although Jane felt comfortable leaving Henry alone with Stretch, we maintained conservative safety measures wherein members of the research team were always present during any interactions with Stretch.

8.2.6.2 Usability and workload

We used the System Usability Scale (SUS) for a global assessment of both pre- and post-use to evaluate general usability. The NASA-TLX provided perceptions of workload for different tasks for both Henry and Jane. These measures are described in Chapter 7. These assessments proved useful to the team for identifying situations in which Stretch was creating user burden and hence targets of opportunity for redesign. For example, the cycle of evaluation revealed a high workload involved in the control of the robot for both Henry and Jane. Improved versions after each design iteration allowed them to operate Stretch with a minimal workload. During one set of tests, the workload involved in controlling the robot was reduced in the aggregated NASA-TLX score by 50% for Henry and by 30% for Jane after the final evaluation. This workload reduction was made possible by developing software that allowed them to predefine complex robot movements that could be executed in real time.

8.2.6.3 Trust

As discussed in Chapter 7, trust in robots should be measured in a multifactorial way to capture perceptions of trust for different tasks (using a rating scale), reasons for trust perceptions (through semistructured interviews), and objectively (through use of the robot). We included these different measures (see Olatunji et al., 2023), and the results provide valuable insights about the

Henry's Trust Ratings and Opinions

Willingness to rely on Stretch to perform task autonomously:
(1=not willing; 5=willing)

Task	Rating
Social participation (game)	5
Docking Stretch	5
Meal preparation and clean up	4
Putting washcloth into laundry	4
Self-feeding	3
Scratching itches	3
Turning on/off a light switch	3
Adjusting blinds	1

Would you be willing to trust the robot to perform self-feeding?
"Arm tasks are 100% predictable but tasks using the automated base movements are 100% random"

Would you be willing to continue to use the robot for adjusting blinds?
"We never even tried this autonomously; too delicate"

Jane's Trust Ratings and Opinions

Willingness to rely on Stretch to perform task autonomously:
(1=not willing; 5=willing)

Task	Rating
Physical exercise	5
Meal preparation	5
Household cleaning	5
Meal preparation	5
Social participation with care recipient	5

Would you be willing to trust the robot to perform these tasks ?
"Yes! it was effective for each and cut down on the time I would have spent doing these tasks"

Would you be willing to continue to use the robot for this task?
"Yes! Can't say no to a robot when it comes around to help!"

FIGURE 8.5
Trust ratings and opinions.

complexity of trust in an assistive robot. Figure 8.5 shows the post-use trust ratings for different tasks as well as quotes from the interviews.

The combination of quantitative ratings and qualitative interview data provides insights into the reasoning for the trust perceptions. In addition, these data illustrate the value of measuring trust for a range of tasks. Such assessments can guide design iterations that are task specific.

8.2.7 Participatory design example

The example of the percussion vest machine provides a compelling illustration of participatory design. The purpose of this machine is to loosen mucus in the lungs. It should be used several times per day but is unfortunately very loud. Henry wanted to be able to turn it on and off by himself so he could do the treatments at a time that was convenient for him and not disruptive to other activities. However, the machine had an on/off button that could not be manipulated by the Stretch grippers. How might Stretch interact with this other technology? As illustrated in Figure 8.6, Henry came up with an idea for a tool that could be held by Stretch to achieve the goal. One of the engineers mocked it up using a computer aided drawing program and produced a prototype using a 3D printer. The occupational therapist added some features to the prototype, and the team iterated on the best angle for pressing the button. After a series of iterations, they had created an effective tool.

This example highlights the importance of the team approach and the value of the active engagement of the end user in the design process. The research team would not have identified this as an important task but clearly it was

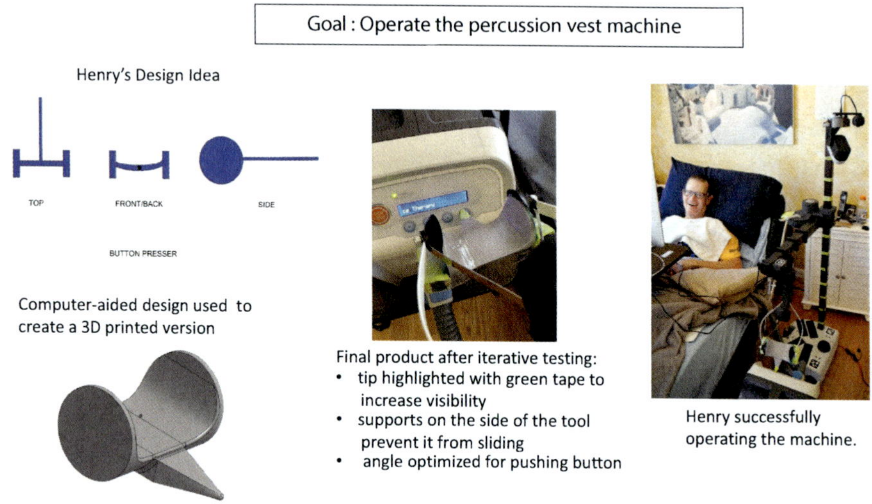

FIGURE 8.6
Participatory design example.

important to Henry. Moreover, enabling Stretch to utilize a tool enhanced its functional abilities.

8.2.8 Ethical considerations

Deploying a robot into a home to support caregiving needs of a person with severe disabilities evokes several of the ethical considerations discussed in Chapter 6. Although the case study presented herein was in the context of a controlled research study with approval from an Institutional Review Board, there are nevertheless ethical issues that can arise. Moreover, as robots become more pervasive in homes, these issues must be addressed. We discuss those most relevant to the caregiving context here (see also recommended reading by Borenstein & Pearson, 2012). The key is to think about the trade-offs between benefits and costs, as well as how having a robot in the home might positively or negatively affect the lives of people in the home (those who live there, work there, or visit there).

Especially because Stretch has several cameras, *privacy* is an issue in this use case. In addition, with the option of teleoperation, Stretch could be controlled from a different room or outside of the home altogether. We need to explore more the use of the different cameras on Stretch and how to convey to people in range that a camera is on at any point in time and who has access to the video information.

Data and access *security* is an issue, generally, in robot design. Henry can store routines, personal preferences, and details about his home. There are various video feeds. The remote connection to the robot must be carefully controlled so that someone without proper training (or with bad intentions) cannot access the Stretch interface. These and other security issues must be considered.

In any caregiving context, the issue of appropriate *trust* will emerge from the perspective of both the care recipient and the care provider. If either user does not trust the robot to perform tasks, it may not be utilized to its full potential. However, over-trust could result in tasks not being completed correctly or safely.

Another issue related to *safety* is that a user might be ready to try the robot for activities before the tasks or tools have been fully tested (i.e., to push the robot to its limits to see how it performs). On the one hand, we might want to allow a person to do what they feel comfortable doing, but, on the other hand, safety issues must always be paramount. This tension is especially an issue for research robots that are still being tested, but the concern will remain when a robot is commercially available and the user is still learning to control it, for example.

An *unintended consequence* discussed in Chapter 6 is that if a robot is providing care for a person, that could result in less human contact and potentially reduce social interactions. In this case study, that was not a major concern, in part because interacting with Stretch increased communication and social interactions between Henry and Jane (using Stretch to enable them to work together) and between Henry and his granddaughter (with Stretch facilitating game-playing). Nevertheless, this should always be a consideration for robots used for providing care.

Another consideration is the *cost/benefit analysis* for different stakeholders, and this is of particular concern in care contexts. We mentioned Henry's Caregiver Principle wherein he would not want to add any assistive device that created more work for Jane, but in general this remains an ethical concern. A caregiver might be hesitant to admit a robot is adding to their caregiver burden if the person believes that the care recipient enjoys having the robot to help them. One important consideration in ethical discussions is that there is seldom a right or a wrong answer. As we emphasized in Chapter 6, the message is of "consideration" – identifying and addressing potential ethical issues is key to reducing harm.

8.3 Lessons learned

- Case studies are invaluable! Of course, we need to extend beyond this case study, but the number of insights we obtained considerably advanced the design of Stretch.
- Think broadly about each stakeholders' needs and involve them in setting up specific goals.

- Be creative in thinking about how to adapt the environment and develop tools that can improve the performance of the robot.
- Conduct preliminary testing prior to field trials to evaluate stability and reliability of the robot in more controlled environments (e.g., production facilities, home simulation labs).
- Recognize the importance of immersion – certain challenges will only become evident when the robot is embedded in an environment and used in natural situations over time.
- Be cognizant of safety issues – research robots should have trained staff always nearby during testing and end users should know how to stop the robot at any time.
- Consider potential ethical issues and address them directly with different stakeholders.
- Iterate, iterate, iterate.
- Robots can change people's lives. In Henry and Jane's words:
- Henry: "Robotics in general have had a very large impact on my life and Stretch is an important link in the evolution of those robotics. Using Stretch was surprisingly easy, showing how adaptable Stretch is."
- Jane: "Robots have influenced Henry's life greatly. They gave him a reason to live...Stretch is the closest to improving Henry's life and therefore mine. We have to ask ourselves over and over, Why robots when a caregiver can do it ten times faster? I see what it does to my husband mentally when he can do things by himself and not depend on anyone."

Recommended readings and links

Readings

Borenstein, J., & Pearson, Y. (2012). Robot caregivers: Ethical issues across the human lifespan. In P. Lin, K. Abney, & G. Bekey (Eds.), *The ethical and social implications of robots* (pp. 251–265). MIT Press.

Kemp, C. C., Edsinger, A., Clever, H. M., & Matulevich, B. (2022). The design of Stretch: A compact, lightweight mobile manipulator for indoor human environments. In *International Conference on Robotics and Automation (ICRA)* (pp. 3150–3157). IEEE.

Nguyen, V., Cakmak, M., Fair-Field, T., Rogers, W. A., & Kemp, C.C. (under review). Beyond motor impairment: Empowering functional performance with robotics. *Occupational Therapy Journal of Research*.

Olatunji, S. A., Nguyen, V., Cakmak, M., Edsinger, A., Kemp, C. C., Rogers, W. A., & Mahajan, H. P. (2024). Immersive participatory design of assistive robots to support older adults. *Ergonomics, 67*, 717–731. https://doi.org/10.1080/00140139.2024.2312529

Olatunji, S. A., Nguyen, V., Cao, Y., Evans, H., Evans, J., Edsinger, A., Kemp, C. C., & Rogers, W. A. (2023). Advancing the design of trustworthy robots for older adults in home environments: A participatory design approach. *Proceedings of the Human Factors and Ergonomics Society Annual Meeting, 67*(1), 2545–2551. https://doi.org/10.1177/21695067231205566

Ranganeni, V., Nguyen, V., Evans, H., Evans, J., Mehu, J., Olatunji, S., Rogers, W., Edsinger, A., Kemp, C., & Cakmak, M. (2024). Robots for humanity: In-home deployment of Stretch RE2. In *ACM/IEEE International Conference on Human-Robot Interaction* (pp. 1299–1301). https://doi.org/10.1145/3610978.3641114

Links

Hello Robot company background:
https://hello-robot.com/about

McKechnie Family LIFE Home:
https://lifehome.ahs.illinois.edu/

Robots for Humanity:
https://r4h.org/

Stretch 3®: A fully integrated mobile manipulator:
https://spectrum.ieee.org/stretch-assistive-robot

This robot could be the key to empowering people with disabilities:
https://hello-robot.com/stretch-3-product

9

Implementation considerations

9.1 Overview of Implementation considerations'

After all the considerations in the foregoing chapters have been addressed, the resulting robot will need to be integrated into the lives of older adults and society. How that will be accomplished is the critical final step – implementation. Just because your robot has been designed with consideration of user needs and is capable of performing tasks reliably and effectively, it will not necessarily be adopted by an individual or by a community.

The Roomba provides an illustrative example. This brand of robotic vacuum has a high market share (estimated as close to 50%) of all robotic vacuums. But in terms of all vacuums sold, robotic vacuums are estimated to be less than 20%. Although these percentages are expected to rise in the future, why is it that robotic vacuums are not more widely used? This is where implementation comes in. Consider an older adult who lives alone and wishes to purchase a robotic vacuum. First, there might be cost considerations, but then there are implementation considerations as well. Will the person be able to get it to work (i.e., set up the programming)? Will it work well on their type of flooring or floorplan? How will it affect the cat and the dog who live in the home? Does it really clean as well as the advertisements suggest (and better than their current method)? There may be privacy and security concerns related to what information is obtained from the home and how it is stored. These and other issues will influence adoption by an individual, which cumulatively will then represent the success of an implementation.

In Chapter 4, we described the primary activities that older adults need to be able to do to function effectively on a daily basis: activities of daily living (ADLs), instrumental ADLs (IADLs), and enhanced ADLs (EADLs). Recently, a new category has been proposed: digital ADLs (DADLs; Mois & Rogers, 2024). Digital technologies and interfaces often require internet access and are dependent on actions by the user to successfully implement them in their day-to-day life. For example, using a smartphone to videochat requires the user to download/access a videochat application, create a user account, and use the application interface to make the call. These activities are prerequisites

DOI: 10.1201/9781032656649-9

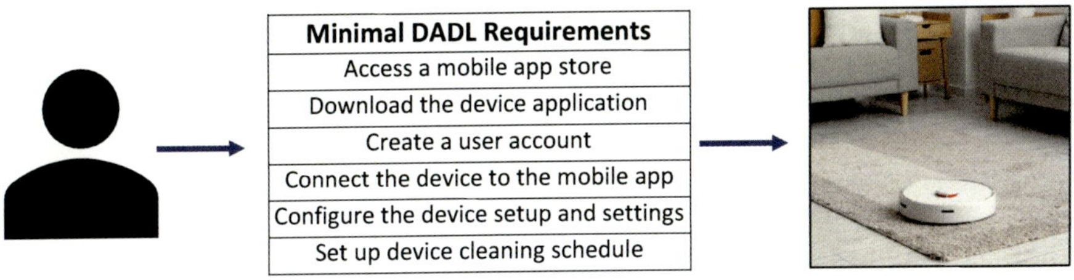

FIGURE 9.1
DADL requirements for implementing a robotic vacuum in the home (from: Mois & Rogers, 2024).

for successfully using digital technologies, and in turn being able to use the devices to accomplish ADLs, IADLs, and EADLs.

Figure 9.1 illustrates the DADL requirements for implementing a robotic vacuum in the home. There are multiple steps required, any one of which might be a barrier to an older adult being able to utilize this technology for the IADL task of housecleaning. For robots that are teleoperated or semiautonomous, where the human is acting as an operator, teammate, or supervisor, the DADL requirements may impose high levels of cognitive, physical, and temporal workload (see Chapter 4). Consequently, the implementation success for a broad range of older adults may be impacted negatively.

The focus of this chapter is on the factors and processes that can increase the likelihood of success or, conversely, decrease the likelihood of failure. We will present established frameworks and models that provide insights into the various aspects of implementation that need to be considered. These theoretical and practical perspectives contextualize the implementation components, identify target users, and clarify potential issues that might arise and need to be addressed. Implementation success will be influenced by the stage of technology development, the traits/characteristics of potential users, their perceptions of the technology, and factors that moderate adoption. We will discuss each of these in turn.

9.2 Technology maturation: the Gartner Hype Cycle

When we think about new technologies and how they are adopted into communities, there are cycles that occur over time. Understanding these trends can guide implementation planning and perhaps temper expectations for success at different points in the cycles. For example, the *Gartner Hype Cycle* provides a graphical representation of the stage of maturation of a given technology. It was developed by Gartner Research (www.gartner.com) to help businesses identify when might be a good time to adopt certain technologies with respect to their strategic goals and likelihood for success. Figure 9.2

depicts the hype cycle for a range of emerging technologies in 2023, with predictions about the future of various technologies, many of which are foundational to the success of robots such as cloud computing, reinforcement learning, and generative artificial intelligence (AI).

Consider the stages of the Gartner Hype Cycle:

- First, there is the *Innovation Trigger*, which is a technological breakthrough that might be mentioned in a media story or described by a start-up company. There may not yet be a viable product or anything commercially viable.
- Second is the *Peak of Inflated Expectations*, where success stories (and failure stories) become prevalent.

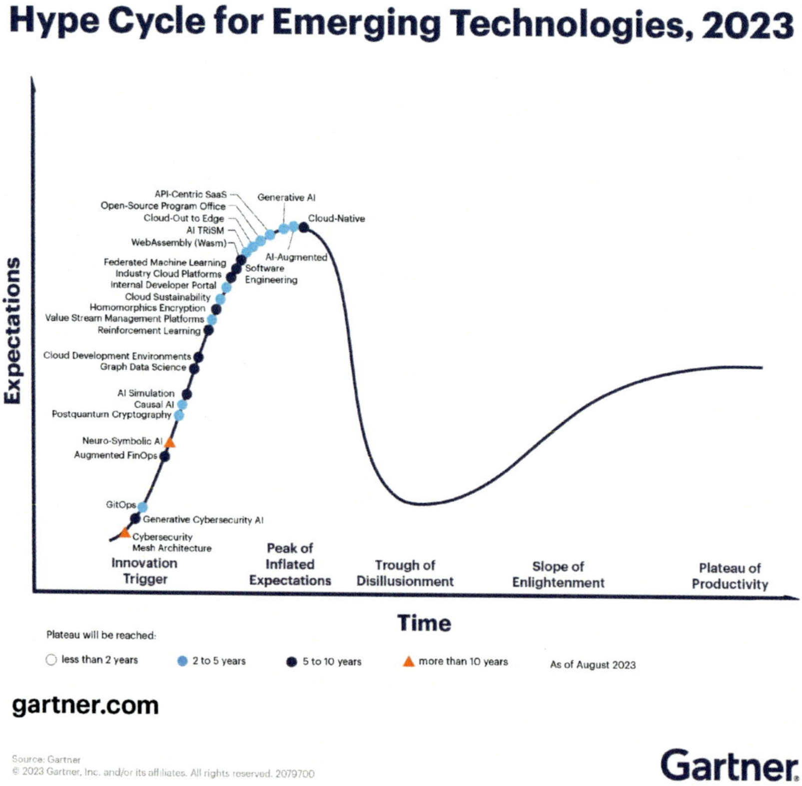

FIGURE 9.2
Gartner Hype Cycle for emerging technologies (from: https://www.gartner.com/en/articles/what-s-new-in-the-2023-gartner-hype-cycle-for-emerging-technologies).

- Third is the *Trough of Disillusionment,* where general interest wanes perhaps because failures outnumber the successes, and the technology does not deliver on its promise.
- Fourth is the *Slope of Enlightenment,* where the benefits of the technology become more evident and later product iterations solve earlier miscues.
- Fifth is the *Plateau of Productivity,* representing mainstream adoption and broad market penetration.

We can use the phases of the hype cycle to make predictions about robots, more specifically. Generally speaking, robots being developed now are in the Innovation Trigger phase. However, there are robots being developed with potential to support older adults with various activities (see Chapters 3 and 4). Specific robots and robot/task combinations will vary in their stage of maturation. For example, robot vacuum cleaners may already be in the Plateau of Productivity, whereas telepresence robots might be in the Slope of Enlightenment, and assistive robots may be in the Peak of Inflated Expectations. (Note that we do not have evidence for these stage attributions; these examples are just illustrative.) Thinking about the stage of maturation of a given robot can inform both the companies developing robots and people and communities contemplating purchasing robots.

9.3 Traits and characteristics of people

In addition to the maturation stage of the technology itself, the rate at which an innovation reaches broad market penetration will be influenced by traits and characteristics of individuals in the target market. The Diffusion of Innovations theoretical framework was developed by a sociologist, Everett Rogers, originally in 1962, to describe how new ideas (i.e., innovations) spread through a population. Although of no relation, one author of this book (Wendy Rogers) remembers being inspired by the keynote address that Everett Rogers gave at the Human Factors and Ergonomics Society (HFES) Annual Meeting in 1997. The meeting was held in Albuquerque, New Mexico, and Everett Rogers was on the faculty at the University of New Mexico. He provided the attendees with an insightful discussion about his diffusion framework. One aspect of the framework was the innovativeness of the adopter (see Figure 9.3).

Rogers (2003) proposed that adopter categories represented idealized groups of individuals that could provide insights about rates of adoption. Depicted in Figure 9.3 are five groups that represent the different rates at which categories of people adopt new innovations:

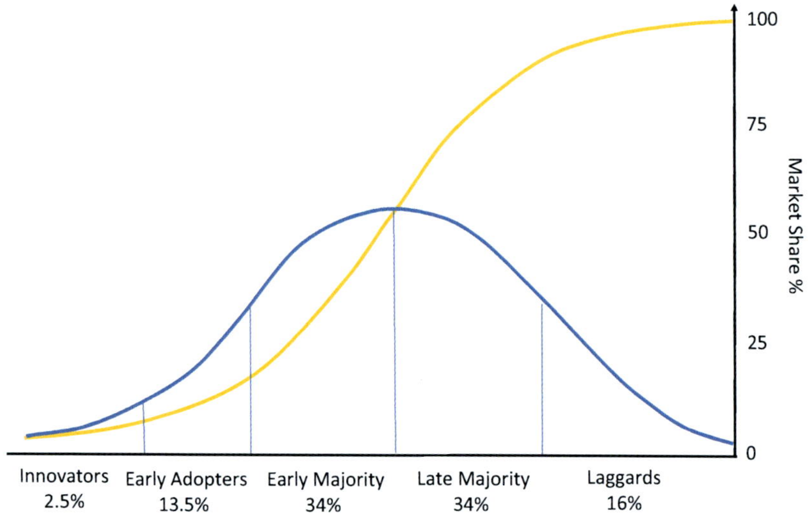

FIGURE 9.3
Diffusion of innovations for different adopter categories (from: Rogers, 2003).

- *Innovators* – this group represents a small percentage of the population. They are willing to take risks on something new, understanding that it might fail. They may have higher incomes making them less susceptible to costs associated with innovation failures.
- *Early Adopters* – this group tends to be well educated, a little more cautious than innovators, but willing to take some risks.
- *Early Majority* – this is a larger group of people who will adopt an innovation after some time has passed and there has been some evidence of success.
- *Late Majority* – a similarly large group but a little slower to adopt and more skeptical. They may adopt out of necessity (when the innovation is so pervasive that they have less choice).
- *Laggards* – this group represents those slowest to adopt an innovation. They may be resistant due to economic resources.

In that same plenary session, the HFES President at the time, Arthur D. Fisk, delivered his address on *Human Factors and the Older Adult* (see Fisk, 1999). This juxtaposition of speeches made clear that the components of Rogers's diffusion of innovations framework should guide human factors thinking about the adoption of new technologies by older adults. As we described in Chapter 2, there is heterogeneity within the older adult segment of the population. There are older adults who are innovators and older adults who are laggards, and everything in between.

9.4 Perceptions about technology

Another important contributor to successful diffusion of an innovation is the innovation itself. Potential adopters will evaluate the innovation with respect to their own current situations. Rogers (2003) described perceived attributes of innovation that drive rates of adoption in a population:

- *Relative Advantage* – is it better than other options, either one's current approach or other new solutions?
- *Compatibility* – does the innovation fit well with one's current situation, values, and needs?
- *Complexity/Simplicity* – is the innovation easy to understand, to learn, and to use?
- *Trialability* – can the person try it out before purchasing or committing to using it?
- *Observability* – are the benefits of the innovation visible or easily conveyed?

We can contextualize these attributes with an example of a socially assistive robot (SAR) meant to provide healthcare reminders, such as for hydration or medication. Considerations might be whether the SAR is better than using an app or an alarm, or perhaps relying on one's spouse for reminders. Will the SAR be functional in the person's home and be able to present the reminders accurately? How difficult will it be to convey to the robot the person's preferred schedule or medication regimen? Can they use the SAR for a while to see if they like it and if it is effective for them? And is it clear that the SAR is serving its purpose and improving their health?

The characteristics can interact and might have different relative weightings. As illustrated in Chapter 8, for a person with limited mobility, the relative advantage of a robot over current methods may be very high, and the person may be willing to invest more time to learn to control it. Designers might think about these different attributes as things to highlight during the implementation of a new robot. For example, how might the relative advantage and the compatibility of a robot be conveyed to a target market? How can the complexity of learning to use it be reduced through design or supported with training? How might people be given a chance to try the robot and/or observe the benefits?

The goal of the diffusion of innovations framework is to represent and understand population-level data and provide valuable categories for consideration. But to predict acceptance *by an individual,* the Technology Acceptance Model (TAM) was proposed by Davis (1989). There have been many adaptations of TAM over time; see Venkatesh et al. (2012) for an integrative review and what they called the UTAUT (Unified Theory of Acceptance and Use of Technology). These general models can be adapted for specific technologies. For example, the Almere model (named after the city Almere, The Netherlands) adapted the UTAUT model to understand robot acceptance by older adults (Heerink et al., 2010) and is depicted in Figure 9.4. Technology acceptance can be measured as intention to use as well as by actual use (also referred to as adoption).

The specific image depicted in Figure 9.4 is from a scoping review that explored the utility of the Almere model (and thus the UTAUT model) for understanding acceptance of social robots for older adults and people with dementia in nursing homes. Felding et al. (2023) found 26 primary articles on acceptance of social robots in nursing homes. They depicted the most studied constructs in green, followed next by orange, then yellow; the constructs colored red were rarely studied in the context they were exploring.

Trust and intention to use were the least directly studied constructs, though that might be an artifact of the context of the research reviewed. Most studied in the context of acceptance of social robots in nursing homes were perceived usefulness, perceived ease of use, and perceived enjoyment. In addition to perceptions, there were potential moderating factors (e.g., age, sex, experience, voluntariness), social influence, and facilitating conditions that were important contributors to robot acceptance by older adults.

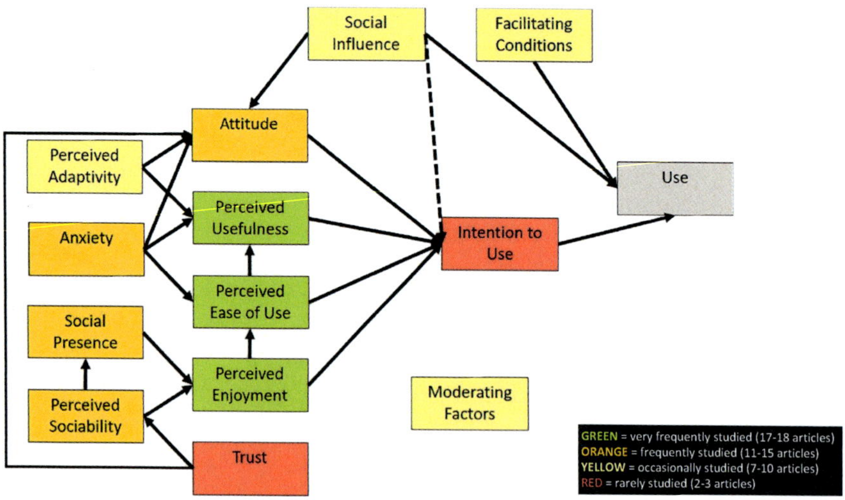

FIGURE 9.4
Almere model (from: originally in Heerink et al., 2010, colored to reflect the scoping review results in Felding et al., 2023).

Social influence refers to whether people in your social sphere are encouraging you to use the technology. Healthcare providers, family members, or peers might encourage an older person to use a robot. In addition are facilitating conditions, which represent the technical and organizational infrastructure necessary for using the robot. Such conditions can include resources, training, and social support for learning to use a robot. For example, instructional support is especially important to enable older adults the opportunity to become comfortable with the robot and confident in their ability to interact with it and to use it for its intended purpose. The category of facilitating conditions relates to issues of maintenance to which we turn next.

9.5 Robot maintenance

What happens if the robot does not work as intended? If an older adult has a robot in their home to assist them with ADL, IADLs, or EADLs, and they have come to rely on that robot, what are their options if it becomes less reliable or stops working altogether?

Robots in a home may require regular maintenance (e.g., cleaning sensors, updating software, calibrating end effectors), and it is unlikely that most older users will be willing or able to perform such maintenance tasks. Moreover, that would be adding to their workload, rather than making their lives easier. Robots in facilities may require more frequent maintenance due to high rates of use. Will robot experts have to be on staff to service the robots? Or will that be the responsibility of the company that sold the robot?

There are likely to be different models that emerge over time as robots become more prevalent in the marketplace. One analogy may be to a furnace where some companies produce the technology, but other companies conduct periodic inspections and perform maintenance tasks. An alternative approach would be analogous to a home security system where the company owns the technology, and the user pays a monthly fee that includes upgrades and maintenance as needed. A third option is akin to appliances such as dishwashers or washing machines where they are purchased and used; if they break, an appliance repair person is called in (who can service various brands, different appliance categories, and a range of repair needs).

Given that home robots represent a new category of technology, there are likely to be other maintenance models as well. Essentially, maintenance issues must be considered in the context of implementation. Individuals, families, communities, and organizations are going to need assurance that the robots they come to rely upon will be available when they are needed. Otherwise, broad scale adoption will not happen.

9.6 Planning and evaluating success

The reach, effectiveness, adoption, implementation, and maintenance (RE-AIM) framework was developed to guide planning and evaluation of programs according to five key outcome variables: reach, effectiveness, adoption, implementation, and maintenance (see Figure 9.5). The goal is to assess barriers to implementation success and encourage people at different levels of a system (e.g., program planners, evaluators, funders, policymakers) to attend to the specific elements that can improve the sustainable implementation of effective interventions that are evidence-based and will be generalizable.

The RE-AIM framework was originally developed to encourage consistent reporting of results from program evaluations. However, it has evolved

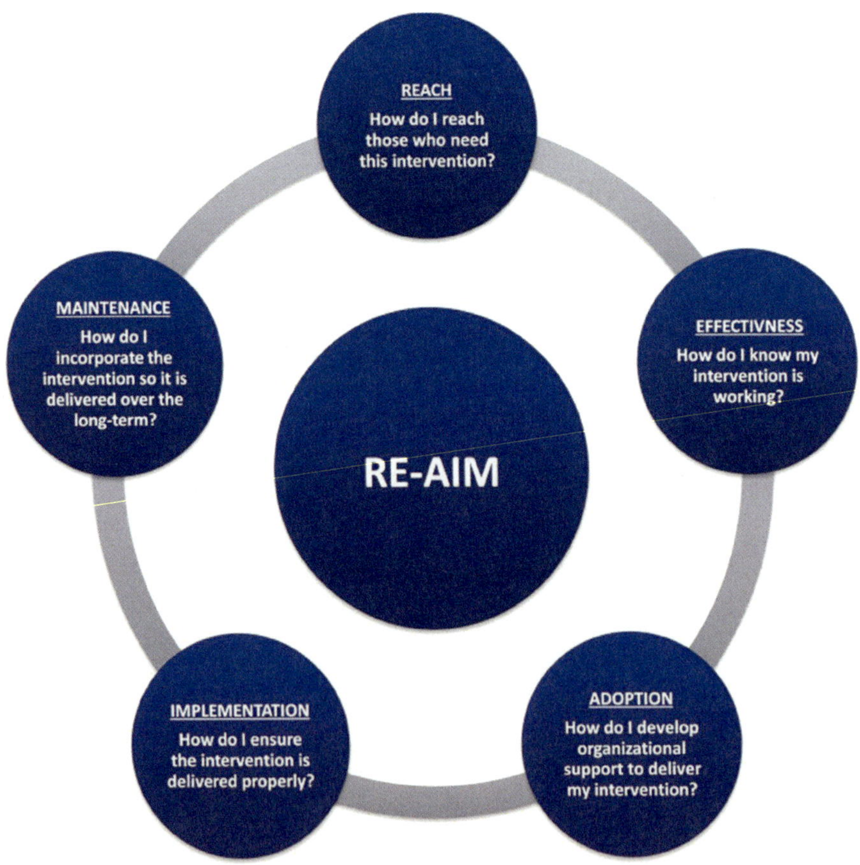
REACH
How do I reach those who need this intervention?
EFFECTIVNESS
How do I know my intervention is working?
ADOPTION
How do I develop organizational support to deliver my intervention?
IMPLEMENTATION
How do I ensure the intervention is delivered properly?
MAINTENANCE
How do I incorporate the intervention so it is delivered over the long-term?
RE-AIM

FIGURE 9.5
RE-AIM elements for planning and evaluating questions (from: Ory et al., 2015).

to be a valuable tool not only for program evaluation but also for planning implementation protocols, interpreting results, and guiding funding as well as policy decisions. There are five key elements:

- *Reach* – engagement of the target population
- *Effectiveness* – positive impact
- *Adoption* – use of the program
- *Implementation* – consistency of delivery and feasibility
- *Maintenance* – sustenance of benefits over time

Consider a robot intended to be used to conduct wellness checks for the residents of a continuing care retirement community (CCRC; as described in Chapter 5). The robot might conduct a series of tasks in the morning such as deliver a newspaper, verify the resident is up and about, and provide individualized reminders for daily activities. In terms of *reach,* the goal might be to support all the older adults living in the community. However, evaluations might reveal that only the higher cognitively functioning older adults tended to interact with the robot, but the lower cognitively functioning individuals did not. Such a finding would provide insights for next steps to either improve the robot design or enhance the facilitating conditions for using the robot. With respect to *effectiveness,* wellness checks are the primary benefit that should be measured. Negative outcomes might be robot-related (someone's room is missed, or incorrect reminders are presented) or person-related (the resident gets annoyed at the robot or does not trust the information being presented). For *adoption,* the interaction environments will need to be considered (e.g., different types of apartments, number of people; see Chapter 5) as well as the potential demands on staff as operators/teammates/supervisors/bystanders (see Chapter 3). *Implementation* would relate to consistency of the robot successfully conducting wellness checks every day for all residents, how it was adapted (or could be) to individual preferences, the cost of the implementation (in terms of the robot(s) but also staff time), and the contributing factors that need to be considered for further implementation efforts. The *maintenance* considerations relate to planning operations (e.g., whether all residents start receiving robot check-ins on the same day or the process be introduced gradually), how long each robot will be used, whether the residents continue to engage with the robot over time, and whether will it continue to function reliably.

The RE-AIM website provides valuable resources and tools that can assist projects with their implementation processes (https://re-aim.org/resources-and-tools/). They have presentations about the different components of the framework for explaining the needs to board members, advisors, funders, and policymakers. The site provides checklists and measures that have been validated and examples of how they have been used.

9.7 Guidelines for implementation

- Consider the DADLs required for using the robot (e.g., access to an app, user account details, device configuration, control needs).
- Identify the stage of maturation of the technology. Is the robot ready for use outside of controlled settings? What are the expectations of people in the target market?
- Recognize that there are categories of adopters. Implementation strategies may need to differ for innovators versus the later majority, for example.
- Highlight the attributes of the technology such as relative advantage, compatibility, and simplicity. Provide opportunities for trying the robot and make benefits of use clear.
- Recognize that perceptions of usefulness, ease of use, and enjoyment will influence intentions to use a robot initially, as well as continued use.
- Capitalize on the potential of social influence to encourage people to use a robot.
- Ensure that facilitating conditions are in place to support use, such as resources and social support during use. Provide appropriate instructional support.
- Set up a maintenance plan to ensure the robot remains functioning, reliable, and safe.
- Utilize the RE-AIM framework for planning and evaluating the introduction of a robot to a person, community, or organization. Consider reach, effectiveness, adoption, implementation, and maintenance.

Recommended readings and links

Readings

Czaja, S. J., & Sharit, J. (2012). *Designing training and instructional programs for older adults*. CRC Press.

Felding, S. A., Koh, W. Q., Teupen, S., Budak, K. B., Uribel, F. L., & Roes, M. (2023). A scoping review using the Almere Model to understand factors facilitating and hindering the acceptance of social robots in nursing homes. *International Journal of Social Robotics, 15*, 1115–1153. https://doi.org/10.1007/s12369-023-01012-1

Glasgow, R. E., & Estabrooks, P. E. (2018). Pragmatic applications of RE-AIM for health care initiatives in community and clinical settings. *Preventing Chronic Disease, 15*, E02. https://doi.org/10.5888/pcd15.170271

Heerink, M., Kröse, B., Evers, V., & Wielinga, B. (2010). Assessing acceptance of assistive social agent technology by older adults: The Almere model. *International Journal of Social Robotics, 2*(4), 361–375. https://doi.org/10.1007/s12369-010-0068-5

Mois, G., & Rogers, W. A. (2024). Developing a framework for digital activities of daily living. *The Gerontologist, 64*(10), gnae110. https://doi.org/10.1093/geront/gnae110

Ory, M. G., Altpeter, M., Belza, B., Helduser, J., Zhang, C., & Smith, M. L. (2015). Perceived utility of the RE-AIM framework for health promotion/disease prevention initiatives for older adults: A case study from the U.S. evidence-based disease prevention initiative. *Frontiers in Public Health,* 2(143). https://doi.org/10.3389/fpubh.2014.00143

Rogers, E. M. (2003). *Diffusion of innovations* (5th ed.). Simon & Schuster.

Links

RE-AIM: Improving Public Health Relevance and Population Health Impact:
https://re-aim.org/

Gartner research:
https://www.gartner.com/en

10

Conclusions

10.1 Potential of robots to improve quality of life for older adults

Robots have tremendous potential to improve quality of life for older adults. The goal of this book was to distill our combined 50+ years of experience in guiding design for technology to support older adults in their everyday lives. Much of that experience specifically focused on the design of robot technology to support aging because the potential is clear. We have a rapidly growing aging population who will require a wide range of support but who want to maintain as much independence and autonomy as possible. At the same time, we have a rapidly developing robotics industry that will be able to do just that, with the caveat that these robots must be designed with consideration of the various factors that impact human–robot interaction (HRI).

Older adults have support needs that are unique compared to younger adults. These needs must be understood by the younger adults and middle-aged adults who are involved in the design and development of robots to maximize perceptions of ease of use and usefulness, which are important predictors of adoption and long-term use. Older adults have been found to be quite positive and open to the idea of robot supports. However, they do have preferences for aspects of HRI, such as the nature of the tasks for which they want robot assistance. Considering these preferences in the design of robots prior to implementation as well as their needs for support will increase the likelihood of acceptance and long-term adoption.

A theme in this book is the importance of appropriately and accurately defining older adults and aging in general. Older adults are diverse in their interests, abilities, and opinions. Just as individuals from any other age group, they have strengths and weaknesses, as well as gains and losses. We need to counter ageist stereotypes that misrepresent the reality of who older adults are. One effective way to do this is to engage a range of older adults in the design process. We discuss different ways to do this throughout the book. By doing so, developers are more likely to create robots that are useful for and easy to use by older adults.

DOI: 10.1201/9781032656649-10

10.2 Human factors process

We developed the HRI framework (Figure 1.4) according to user-centered and universal design principles. The framework encompasses the four primary dimensions of HRI: the human, the robot, the interaction, and the environment. These dimensions represent the breadth of variables that should be considered in the design of a robot; they are meant to be generally representative rather than comprehensive. As such, the framework can be used by robot developers to steer design priorities and specifications, and by researchers to delineate factors that may influence HRI. Our hope is that readers of this book use this framework for each development or research project as a starting point. They should look beyond the framework as well to understand any factors that might be unique to their particular users, robots, settings, or applications.

Robots have been created in a wide range of shapes, sizes, and categories. We discussed a range of robot categories including assistive, exoskeleton, mobile, social, and telepresence and provided many examples of different types of robots, which were meant to be illustrative rather than comprehensive. We know with the rapid development of robotics that some examples we provided may no longer be available or might not have made it to the marketplace. Nevertheless, the processes we discuss are based in human factors and represent the gold standard for design. Therefore, the framework and processes we provided can and should be applied to future robots and applications.

10.3 Applying the guidelines in the design process

The process we have recommended is to consider the different dimensions of the HRI framework and use this information to guide design and deployment.

- Determine who will be using the robot.
- Identify their needs and how the robot might meet those needs.
- Specify the requirements for the robot design.
- Decide what task(s) will be performed by the human and the robot.
- Define the interaction context (e.g., indoors/outdoors, multiple people in the area, need for integration with other technology).

By bringing awareness and attention to the range of factors that can impact older adults and HRI and providing a process to follow, our intention is that robots will be developed that are more useful and usable by the intended

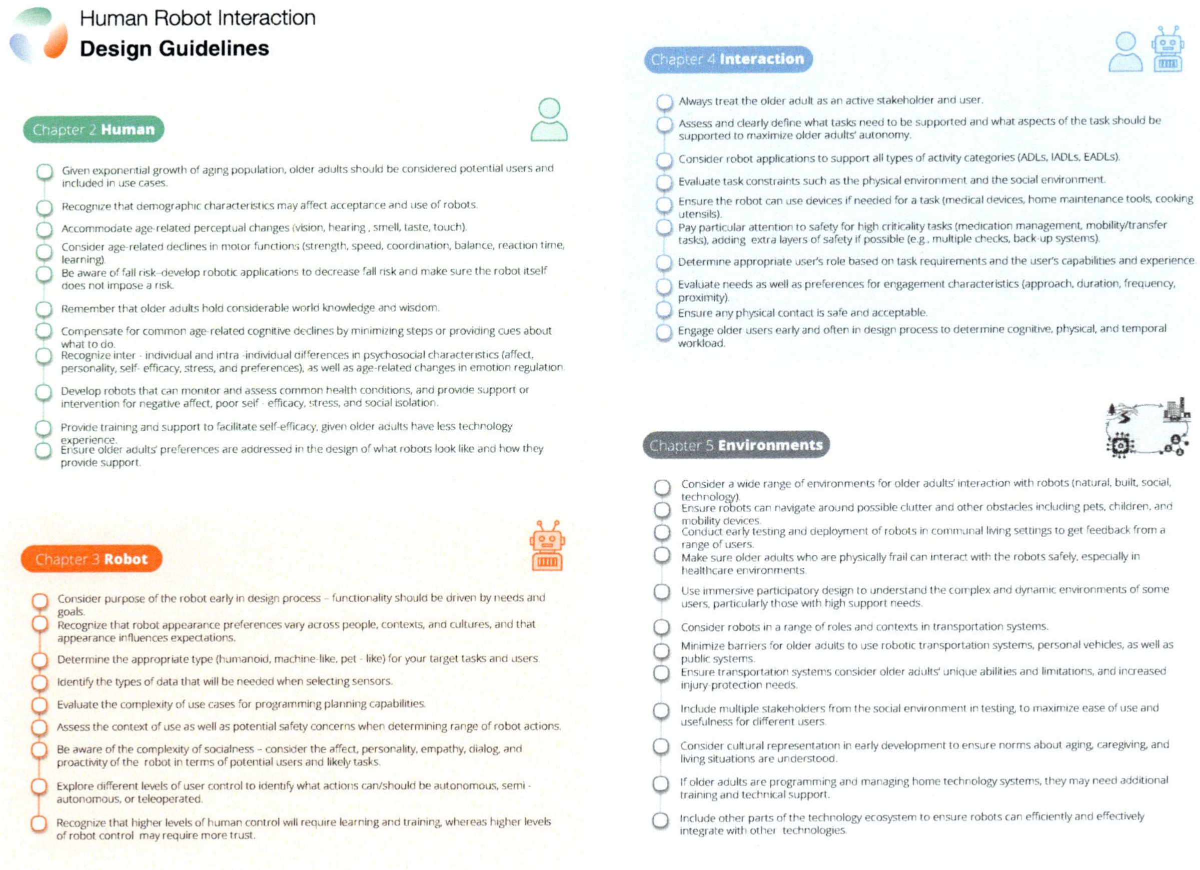

FIGURE 10.1
HRI design guidelines (Recommend printing as 36 × 24-inch poster).

Chapter 6 **Ethics**

- Clearly define problems, solutions, and relevant stakeholders who might be affected by introduction of robot.
- Review ethical topics to identify relevance for each HRI situation.
- Explore different dimensions of situations and perspectives of various stakeholders.
- Develop priorities to guide decision making (maximize autonomy of the person, minimize harm).
- Consider consequences of different design decisions.
- Ensure transparency of robot decisions and actions so the human understands the reasons
- Conduct failure mode and effects analysis for the robot and human error analysis for the person to identify - and mitigate – safety risks.
- Attend to physical safety risks as well as emotional and mental health risks.
- Iteratively review potential ethical issues at different stages (idea conception →market introduction).
- Consider ethical issues related to well - being, care practices, and justice.

Chapter 7 **Methods and Measures**

- Consider the range of stakeholders that should be represented in assessments.
- Design evaluation materials to be accessible to people with different abilities and disabilities.
- Use personas to gain insights about older adults' specific needs, goals, preferences, and everyday activities and behaviors.
- Involve older adults in the design process to the degree possible.
- Carefully select a method for demonstrating a robot's capabilities; consider whether to show ideal or realistic behavior.
- Use questionnaires to collect data when specific questions and potential response categories are known.
- Use interviews to collect rich details and contextual understanding of attitudes and behaviors.
- Conduct interviews with subject matter experts when starting research in new field or with new population.
- When designing interaction studies, consider whether to control the context or environment and whether to control or measure the behavior of the robot.
- Consider timing of HRI measures; whether measures should be administered one time or both pre - and post - interaction.

Chapter 8 **Lessons Learned**

- Case studies are invaluable!
- Think broadly about each stakeholders' needs and involve them in setting up specific goals.
- Be creative in thinking about how to adapt the environment and develop tools that can improve the performance of the robot.
- Conduct preliminary testing prior to field trials to evaluate stability and reliability of the robot in more controlled environments.
- Recognize the importance of immersion-certain challenges will only become evident when the robot is embedded in an environment and used in natural situations over time.
- Be cognizant of safety issues-research robots should have trained staff always nearby during testing and end users should know how to stop the robot at any time.
- Consider potential ethical issues and address them directly with different stakeholders.
- Iterate, iterate, iterate.
- Robots can change people's lives!

Chapter 9 **Implementaion**

- Consider the digital activities of daily living required for using the robot.
- Identify the stage of maturation of the technology. Is the robot ready for use outside of controlled settings? What are the expectations of people in the target market?
- Recognize that there are categories of adopters. Implementation strategies may need to differ for innovators versus the later majority, for example.
- Highlight the attributes of the technology such as relative advantage, compatibility, and simplicity. Provide opportunities for trying the robot and make benefits of use clear.
- Recognize that perceptions of usefulness, ease of use, and enjoyment will influence intentions to use a robot initially, as well as continued use.
- Capitalize on the potential of social influence to encourage people to use a robot.
- Ensure that facilitating conditions are in place to support use, such as resources and social support during use.
- Set up a maintenance plan to ensure the robot remains functioning, reliable, and safe.
- Utilize the RE-AIM framework for planning and evaluating the introduction of a robot to a person, community, or organization.

FIGURE 10.1
(Continued)

users. At the end of most chapters, we present actionable guidelines intended as "news you can use." We have compiled a summary of these guidelines in Figure 10.1. We suggest printing these compiled guidelines along with the framework (Figure 1.4) to use as a reference and checklist throughout the design and development process.

We discussed a range of useful HRI design methods and assessment measures and provided examples of how they have been used. We aimed to include information that would be relevant to developers as well as researchers. The user-centered design approaches range from using personas, to questionnaire methods, to participatory immersive design methods. The recommended measures include those focused on acceptance, trust, attitudes, preferences, experience, usability, as well as more general measures. Together these methods and measures for evaluating different aspects of HRI can bring attention to barriers and facilitators of successful adoption of robots to support older adults.

In our experience, even well-intentioned developers can face ethical dilemmas in designing robots for older adults, from unintendedly biased algorithms to controversial data collection policies to gaps in understanding older adults' needs or preferences. Should a robot collect data about an older adult without their knowledge if it enables the robot to prevent an injury or save their life? Who decides what data will be collected, who can access and use that data, and how these practices should be communicated to the user?

Ethics should be a fundamental part of technology design, not a specialty to apply when ethical issues arise. A former student in our lab who is now an expert in technology and ethics, Dr. Casey Fiesler explains the importance of engaging in a foundational ethics practice in a video (https://www.youtube.com/watch?v=ZcbpT4ESTmA), emphasizing the need to be critical and concerned about unintended negative outcomes. She states that this perspective does not reflect an anti-technology view, but rather

> if we want technology like AI to do good for the world, to be the best that it can possibly be, it is incredibly important that we have foresight about potential harms and also that we learn from the past [ethical controversies].

We share this view and encourage developers to consider potential ethical implications throughout the entire design process.

10.4 Systemic supports needed

The title of this book is *Designing Robots to Improve Quality of Life for Older Adults*. However, it will take more than designing robots well to improve the lives of older adults as a whole. We discussed potential challenges to implementing robots. Successful implementation means that robots will be integrated into the lives of older adults and society. To improve the lives of all older adults, robots will need to be integrated into (and supported by) the societal infrastructure.

In 2017, we published a paper (Rogers & Mitzner, 2017) entitled "Envisioning the future for older adults: Autonomy, health, well-being, and social connectedness with technology support," in the journal *Futures* as part of a special issue on "Envisioning Inclusive Futures." The goal of our paper was to envision the future of older adults in the year 2050. We expected – and still do – that robots would play a pivotal role in supporting older adults and their needs. Even in the relatively short time since we published that paper, we have seen a lot of advancements in robot development and the underlying technological foundations (e.g., sensors, generative artificial intelligence [AI], voice recognition). Robots are appearing in public spaces such as hotels, hospitals, and grocery stores. There are robots that are commercially available as we have described throughout the book. Nevertheless, there is much more to be done before we will see widespread adoption of robots that support the health and wellness of older adults in their living environments.

Societal factors can facilitate (or impede) the uptake of robots in the lives of older adults. For example, facilitators at the societal level might include insurance coverage of assistive robots and healthcare robots and infrastructure to enable professional caregivers to utilize robots (e.g., through technology literacy or instructional support). The diversity of older adults and their needs must be accommodated as this segment of the population will continue to grow in upcoming years. Broad issues of cost and access are relevant with robots, as with other advanced technologies, to minimize digital inequities. Specific impediments to the uptake of robots are myriad and potentially difficult to predict. Social stigma around using a robot may be a factor. Privacy concerns, cost issues, safety concerns, negative perceptions about robots, and so on may all play a role in the rate of robot adoption by older adults.

Public policy must be developed to support robot development and implementation, including providing oversight when necessary to ensure robot developers are adhering to established laws and regulations. Privacy and security standards need to be developed to protect the autonomy of older adults if they choose to adopt robots in their daily lives. Liability and responsibility determinations will be needed as well. These and other policy considerations are beyond the scope of our book, but we have provided relevant recommended readings and links.

10.5 Conclusion

Robots, in their many forms, have the potential to improve quality of life for older adults. The information we have presented provides guidance for the design process. We emphasize the word *process*. There is a process for understanding needs, engaging end users, iteratively designing/redesigning based on user feedback, considering ethical issues, and developing the facilitating conditions for successful implementation. Our goal was to provide a roadmap and resource guide to support the process.

Recommended readings and links

Readings

Mintrom, M., Sumartojo, S., Kulić, D., Tian, L., Carreno-Medrano, P., & Allen, A. (2021). Robots in public spaces: Implications for policy design. *Policy Design and Practice, 5*(2), 123–139. https://doi.org/10.1080/25741292.2021.1905342

Rogers, W. A., & Mitzner, T. L. (2017). Envisioning the future for older adults: Autonomy, health, well-being, and social connectedness with technology support. *Futures, 87*, 133–139. https://doi.org/10.1016/j.futures.2016.07.002

Links

AI ethics series – AI and ethical debt with Casey Fiesler:
https://www.youtube.com/watch?v=ZcbpT4ESTmA

How humans respond to robots: Building public policy through good design:
https://www.brookings.edu/articles/how-humans-respond-to-robots-building-public-policy-through-good-design

Bibliography

Chapter 1

Balaguer, C., Giménez, A., Jardón, A., Correal, R., Cabas, R., & Staroverov, P. (2003). Light weight autonomous climbing robot for elderly and disabled persons' services. *Field and Service Robotics, Recent Advances in Research and Applications*, FSR 2003, Lake Yamanaka, Japan. https://doi.org/10.1007/10991459_39

Beer, J. M., Prakash, A., Smarr, C.-A., Chen, T. L., Hawkins, K., Nguyen, H., Deyle, T., Mitzner, T. L., Kemp, C. C., & Rogers, W. A. (2017). Older users' acceptance of an assistive robot: Attitudinal changes following brief exposure. *Gerontechnology, 16*(1), 21–36. https://doi.org/10.4017/gt.2017.16.1.003.00

Gasteiger, N., Loveys, K., Law, M., & Broadbent, E. (2021). Friends from the future: A scoping review of research into robots and computer agents to combat loneliness in older people. *Clinical Interventions in Aging, 16,* 941–971. https://doi.org/10.2147/cia.s282709

Rogers, W. A., & Mitzner, T. L. (2017). Human-robot interaction for older adults. In P. A. Laplante (Ed.), *Encyclopedia of computer science and technology* (2nd ed., pp. 1–11). Taylor & Francis.

Schaefer, K. E., Adams, J. K., Cook, J. G., Bardwell-Owens, A., & Hancock, P. A. (2015). The future of robotic design: Trends from the history of media representations. *Ergonomics in Design, 23*(1), 13–19. https://doi.org/10.1177/1064804614562214

Stuck, R. E., & Rogers, W. A. (2018). Older adults' perceptions of supporting factors of trust in a robot care provider. *Journal of Robotics, 2018,* 1–11. https://doi.org/10.1155/2018/6519713

Wiczorek, R., Bayles, M. A., & Rogers, W. A. (2020). Domestic robots for older adults: Design approaches and recommendations. In L. Moody, A. Woodcock, D. McDonagh, & L. C. Jain (Eds.), *Design of assistive technology for ageing populations* (pp. 203–219). Springer. https://doi.org/10.1007/978-3-030-26292-1_11

Chapter 2

Beer, J. M., Prakash, A., Smarr, C.-A., Chen, T. L., Hawkins, K., Nguyen, H., Deyle, T., Mitzner, T. L., Kemp, C. C., & Rogers, W. A. (2017). Older users' acceptance of an assistive robot: Attitudinal changes following brief exposure. *Gerontechnology, 16,* 21–36. https://doi.org/10.4017/gt.2017.16.1.003.00

Boot, W., Charness, N., Czaja, S. J., & Rogers, W. A. (2020). *Designing for older adults: Case studies, methods, and tools* (1st ed.). CRC Press.

Centers for Medicare & Medicaid Services (2021). *Medicare chronic condition charts.* Chronic Conditions Warehouse (CCW). https://www.cms.gov/data-research/research/statistical-resources-dually-eligible-beneficiaries/data-tools-researchers

Chen, T. L., Bhattacharjee, T., Beer, J. M., Ting, L. H., Hackney, M. E., Rogers, W. A., & Kemp, C. (2017). Older adults' acceptance of a robot for partner dance-based exercise. *PLoS One 12*(10), e0182736.

Czaja, S. J., Boot, W. R., Charness, N., & Rogers, W. A. (2019). *Designing for older adults: Principles and creative human factors approaches* (3rd ed.). CRC Press.

Czaja, S. J., & Sharit, J. (2012). *Designing training and instructional programs for older adults* (1st ed.). CRC Press.

McLaughlin, A., & Pak, R. (2020). *Designing displays for older adults* (2nd ed.). CRC Press.

Mitzner, T. L., Tiberio, L., Kemp, C. C., & Rogers, W. A. (2018). Understanding health-care providers' perceptions of a personal assistant robot. *Gerontechnology, 17,* 48–55. https://doi.org/10.4017/gt.2018.17.1.005.00

Prakash, A., & Rogers, W. A. (2015). Why some humanoid faces are perceived more positively than others: Effects of human-likeness and task. *International Journal of Social Robotics, 7,* 309–331.

Smarr, C.-A., Mitzner, T. L., Beer, J. M., Prakash, A., Chen, T. L., Kemp, C. C., & Rogers, W. A. (2014). Domestic robots for older adults: Attitudes, preferences, and potential. *International Journal of Social Robotics, 6*(2), 229–247.

Trifilio, E., Williamson, J. B., & Heilman, K. M. (2020). Changes in emotions and mood with aging. In K. M. Heilman & S. E. Nadeau (Eds.), *Cognitive changes and the aging brain* (pp. 127–139). Cambridge University Press.

UN DESA (2023). *World social report 2023: Leaving no one behind in an ageing world.* https://social.desa.un.org/publications/undesa-world-social-report-2023

Chapter 3

Bayles, M. A., Lee, J., Kadylak, T., & Rogers, W. A. (2023). Understanding older adults' initial perceptions of robot appearance and function: Implications for acceptance. *Gerontechnology, 22.* https://doi.org/10.4017/gt.2023.22.2.bay.08

Beer, J. M., Fisk, A. D., & Rogers, W. A. (2014). Toward a framework for levels of robot autonomy in human-robot interaction. *Journal of Human-Robot Interaction, 3,* 74–99. PMCID: PMC5656240

Beer, J. M., Prakash, A., Smarr, C.-A., Chen, T. L., Hawkins, K., Nguyen, H., Deyle, T., Mitzner, T. L., Kemp, C. C., & Rogers, W. A. (2017). Older users' acceptance of an assistive robot: Attitudinal changes following brief exposure. *Gerontechnology, 16,* 21–36. PMCID: PMC6554728.

Beer, J. M., Smarr, C.-A., Fisk, A. D., & Rogers, W. A. (2015). Younger and older users' recognition of virtual agent facial expressions. *International Journal of Human-Computer Studies, 57,* 1–20.

Goetz, J. Kiesler, S., & Powers, A. (2003). Matching robot appearance and behavior to tasks to improve human-robot cooperation. *The 12th IEEE International*

Workshop on Robot and Human Interactive Communication Proceedings: ROMAN 2003 (pp. 55–60). https://doi.org/10.1109/ROMAN.2003.1251796

Kadylak, T., Bayles, M. A., & Rogers, W. A. (2023). Are friendly robots trusted more? An analysis of robot sociability and trust. *Robotics, 12*, 162. https://doi.org/10.3390/robotics12060162

Leng, M, Liu, P., Zhang, P., Hu, M., Zhou, H., Li, G., Yin, H., & Chen, L. (2019). Pet robot intervention for people with dementia: A systematic review and meta-analysis of randomized controlled trials. *Psychiatry Research, 271*, 516–525. https://doi.org/10.1016/j.psychres.2018.12.032

Li, D., Rau, P. L. P., & Li, Y. (2010). A cross-cultural study: Effect of robot appearance and task. *International Journal of Social Robotics, 2*, 175–186. https://doi.org/10.1007/s12369-010-0056-9

Mori, M. (1970). The uncanny valley. *Energy 7(4)*, 33–35 (translated into English by K. F. MacDorman & T. Minato, 2005, *Proceedings of the Humanoids-2005 workshop: Views of the uncanny valley*).

Prakash, A., & Rogers, W. A. (2015). Why some humanoid faces are perceived more positively than others: Effects of human-likeness and task. *International Journal of Social Robotics, 7*, 309–331.

Sheridan, T. B., & Parasuraman, R. (2005). Human-automation interaction. *Reviews of Human Factors and Ergonomics, 1*(1), 89–129. https://doi.org/10.1518/155723405783703082

Sheridan, T. B., & Verplank, W. L. (1978). *Human and computer control of undersea teleoperators* (Man-Machine Systems Lab Report). Massachusetts Institute of Technology.

Sung, J. Y., Grinter, R. E., & Christensen, H. I. (2009). "Pimp my Roomba": Designing for personalization. *CHI '09: Proceedings of the SIGCHI Conference on Human Factors in Computing Systems*, Boston, MA, USA (pp. 193–196).

Van Breemen, A., Yan, X., & Meerbeek, B. (2005). iCat: An animated user-interface robot with personality. *AAMAS '05: Proceedings of the Fourth International Joint Conference on Autonomous Agents and Multiagent Systems* (pp. 143–144). https://doi.org/10.1145/1082473.1082823

Chapter 4

Ajaykumar, G., & Huang, C. M. (2023). Older adults' task preferences for robot assistance in the home. arXiv preprint. https://arxiv.org/abs/2302.12686

Ajaykumar, G., Pineda, K. T., & Huang, C. M. (2023). Older adults' expectations, experiences, and preferences in programming physical robot assistance. *International Journal of Human-Computer Studies, 180*, 103127.

Beer, J. M., Prakash, A., Smarr, C.-A., Mitzner, T. L., Kemp, C. C., & Rogers, W. A. (2012a, September). "Commanding your robot" older adults' preferences for methods of robot control. *Proceedings of the Human Factors and Ergonomics Society Annual Meeting, 56*(1), 1263–1267.

Beer, J. M., Smarr, C.-A., Chen, T. L., Mitzner, T. L., Kemp, C. C., & Rogers, W. A. (2012b). The domesticated robot: Design guidelines for assisting older adults to age in place. *Proceedings of the 7th IEEE/ACM International Conference on Human-Robot Interaction (HRI'12)*, Boston, MA.

Fausset, C. B., Kelly, A. J., Rogers, W. A., & Fisk, A. D. (2011). Challenges to aging in place: Understanding home maintenance difficulties. *Journal of Housing for the Elderly, 25*(2), 125–141. https://doi.org/10.1080/02763893.2011.571105

Kantor, E. D., Rehm, C. D., Haas, J. S., Chan, A. T., & Giovannucci, E. L. (2015). Trends in prescription drug use among adults in the United States from 1999–2012. *JAMA, 314*(17), 1818–1831. https://doi.org/10.1001/jama.2015.13766

Lehdonvirta, V., Shi, L. P., Hertog, E., Nagase, N., & Ohta, Y. (2023). The future(s) of unpaid work: How susceptible do experts from different backgrounds think the domestic sphere is to automation? *PLoS One, 18*(2), e0281282. https://doi.org/10.1371/journal.pone.0281282

Liu, J., Yu, Y., Yan, S., Zeng, Y., Su, S., He, T., Wang, Z., Ding, Q., Zhang, R., Li, W., Wang, X., Zhang, L., & Yue, X. (2023). Risk factors for self-reported medication adherence in community-dwelling older patients with multimorbidity and polypharmacy: A multicenter cross-sectional study. *BMC Geriatrics, 23*(1). https://doi.org/10.1186/s12877-023-03768-7

National Health Interview Survey. (2016). QuickStats: Percentage of adults with activity limitations, by age group and type of limitation, United States, 2014. *Morbidity and Mortality Weekly Report, 65*(1), 14.

New York State Office for the Aging. (2023). *FA's rollout of AI companion robot ElliQ shows 95% reduction in loneliness*. https://aging.ny.gov/news/nysofas-rollout-ai-companion-robot-elliq-shows-95-reduction-loneliness

Nolan, E. (2024). For older people who are lonely, is the solution a robot friend? *The New York Times*. https://www.nytimes.com/2024/07/06/nyregion/ai-robot-elliq-loneliness.html

Rogers, W. A., Mitzner, T. L., & Bixter, M. T. (2020). Understanding the potential of technology to support enhanced activities of daily living (EADLs). *Gerontechnology, 19*(2), 125–137.

Savage, N. (2022). Robots rise to meet the challenge of caring for old people. *Nature, 601*(7893), S8–S10. https://doi.org/10.1038/d41586-022-00072-z

Smarr, C.-A., Mitzner, T. L., Beer, J. M., Prakash, A., Chen, T. L., Kemp, C. C., & Rogers, W. A. (2014). Domestic robots for older adults: Attitudes, preferences, and potential. *International Journal of Social Robotics, 6*, 229–247.

Wolff, J. L., Feder, J., & Schulz, R. (2016). Supporting family caregivers of older Americans. *The New England Journal of Medicine, 375*(26), 2513–2515. https://doi.org/10.1056/NEJMp1612351

Wolinsky, F. D., Bentler, S. E., Hockenberry, J., Jones, M. P., Obrizan, M., Weigel, P. A. M., Kaskie, B., & Wallace, R. B. (2011). Long-term declines in ADLs, IADLs, and mobility among older Medicare beneficiaries. *BMC Geriatrics, 11*, 43.

Chapter 5

Ausubel, J. (2020). *Older people are more likely to live alone in the US than elsewhere in the world*. Pew Research Center. https://www.pewresearch.org/short-reads/2020/03/10/older-people-are-more-likely-to-live-alone-in-the-u-s-than-elsewhere-in-the-world/

Avioz-Sarig, O., Olatunji, S., Sarne-Fleischmann, V., & Edan, Y. (2021). Robotic system for physical training of older adults. *International Journal of Social Robotics 13*, 1109–1124. https://doi.org/10.1007/s12369-020-00697-y

Chen, C., Ding, S., & Wang, J. (2023). Digital health for aging populations. *Nature Medicine, 29*(7), 1623–1630. https://doi.org/10.1038/s41591-023-02391-8

Insurance Institute for Highway Safety (IIHS). (2020). Fatality facts 2022: Older people. Insurance Institute for Highway Safety (IIHS). Available at: https://www.iihs.org/topics/fatality-statistics/detail/older-people

Li, S., Milligan, K., Blythe, P., Zhang, Y., Edwards, S., Palmarini, N., Corner, L., Ji, Y., Zhang, F., & Namdeo, A. (2023). Exploring the role of human-following robots in supporting the mobility and wellbeing of older people. *Scientific Reports, 13*(1), 6512. https://doi.org/10.1038/s41598-023-33837-1

Mitzner, T. L., Chen, T. L., Kemp, C. C., & Rogers, W. A. (2014). Identifying the potential for robotics to assist older adults in different living environments. *International Journal of Social Robotics, 6*(2), 213–227. https://doi.org/10.1007/s12369-013-0218-7

Nagasawa, T., Oyake, K., Kawahara, M., Kaneko, S.-i., & Capi, G. (2022). Development of a walking assistive robot for elderly people in outdoor environments. *2nd International Conference on Image Processing and Robotics (ICIPRob)*, Colombo (pp. 1–5). https://doi.org/10.1109/ICIPRob54042.2022.9798726

Nakagawa, Y., Park, K., Ueda, H., & Ono, H. (2014). Driving assistance with conversation robot for elderly drivers. In C. Stephanidis & M. Antona (Eds.), *Universal access in human-computer interaction. Aging and Assistive Environments. UAHCI 2014. Lecture Notes in Computer Science* (vol. 8515). Heraklion. https://doi.org/10.1007/978-3-319-07446-7_71

Shanahan, D., Bush, R., Gaston, K., Lin, B. B., Dean, J., Barber, E., & Fuller, R. A. (2016). Health benefits from nature experiences depend on dose. *Scientific Reports, 6*, 28551. https://doi.org/10.1038/srep28551

Usmani, U. A., Happonen, A., & Watada, J. (2023). Revolutionizing transportation: Advancements in robot-assisted mobility systems. In M. Tuba, S. Akashe, & A. Joshi (Eds.), *ICT Infrastructure and Computing. ICT4SD 2023. Lecture notes in networks and systems* (vol. 754). Goa. https://doi.org/10.1007/978-981-99-4932-8_55

Wilson, C. M., Boright, L., Louie, W. G., Shahverdi, P., Arena, S. K., Benbow, R., Wilson, J. R., Chen, Q., Rousso, K., & Huang, N. (2023). Effect of robotic delivery of physical activity and fall prevention exercise in older adults: A pilot cohort study. *Cureus, 15*(8), e44264. https://doi.org/10.7759/cureus.44264

Zhao, Q., Chen, Z., Landis, C. D., Lytle, A., Rao, A. K., Zanotto, D., & Guo, Y. (2022). Gait monitoring for older adults during guided walking: An integrated assistive robot and wearable sensor approach. *Wearable Technologies, 3*, e28. https://doi.org/10.1017/wtc.2022.23

Chapter 6

Hare, S. (2021). *Technology is not neutral: A short guide to technology ethics.* London Publishing Partnership.

Koh, W. Q., Vandemeulebroucke, T., Gastmans, C., Miranda, R., & Van den Block, L. (2023). The ethics of pet robots in dementia care settings: Care professionals' and organizational leaders' ethical intuitions. *Frontiers in Psychiatry, 14*, 1052889. https://doi.org/10.3389/fpsyt.2023.1052889

Lin, P., Abney, K., & Bekey, G. (2012). *The ethical and social implications of robots*. MIT Press.

Major, L., & Shah, J. (2020). *What to expect when you're expecting robots*. Basic Books.

Mitzner, T. L., Chen, T. L., Kemp, C. C., & Rogers, W. A. (2014). Identifying the potential for robotics to assist older adults in different living environments. *International Journal of Social Robotics, 6*(2), 213–227.

Sharit, J. (2012). Human error and human reliability analysis. In G. Salvendy (Ed.), *Handbook of human factors and ergonomics* (4th ed., pp. 734–800). Wiley & Sons.

Chapter 7

Bartneck, C., Croft, E., Kulic, D., & Zoghbi, S. (2009). Measurement instruments for the anthropomorphism, animacy, likeability, perceived intelligence, and perceived safety of robots. *International Journal of Social Robotics,* 1(1) 71–81. https://doi.org/10.1007/s12369-008-0001-3

Bayles, M. A., Mitzner, T. L. & Rogers, W. A. (2021). *TechSAge Tool: Conducting research with older adults aging with sensory and mobility disabilities*. Rehabilitation Engineering Research Center on Technologies to Support Aging-in-Place for People with Long-Term Disabilities. https://techsage.gatech.edu/sites/default/files/2022-01/TechSAge%20Tool_ResearchGuide.pdf

Brooke, J. (1996). SUS—A quick and dirty usability scale. *Usability Evaluation in Industry, 189*, 4–7. https://doi.org/10.1201/9781498710411-35

Carpinella, C. M., Wyman, A. B., Perez, M. A., & Stroessner, S. J. (2017). The robotic social attributes scale (RoSAS): Development and validation. *Proceedings of the 2017 ACM/IEEE International Conference on Human-Robot Interaction*, Vienna, Austria.

Desai, M. (2012). *Modeling trust to improve human-robot interaction*. Unpublished doctoral dissertation. University of Massachusetts Lowell.

Hart, S. G. (2006). NASA-task load index (NASA-TLX): 20 years later. *Proceedings of the Human Factors and Ergonomic Society Annual Meeting, 50*, 904–908.

Jian, J. Y., Bisantz, A. M., & Drury, C. G. (2000). Foundations for an empirically determined scale of trust in automated systems. *International Journal of Cognitive Ergonomics, 4*, 53–71. https://doi.org/10.1207/S15327566IJCE0401_04

Kohn, S. C., de Visser, E. J., Wiese, E., Lee, Y. C., & Shaw, T. H. (2021). Measurement of trust in automation: A narrative review and reference guide. *Frontiers in Psychology, 12*, 604977. https://doi.org/10.3389/fpsyg.2021.604977

Körber, M., Gold, C., Goncalves, J., & Bengler, K. (2015). Vertrauen in Automation-Messung, Auswirkung und Einflüsse. *TÜV SÜD Akademie GmbH*, 7.

Laugwitz, B., Held, T., & Schrepp, M. (2008). USAB 2008, LNCS 5298. In Andreas Holzinger (Ed.), P *Construction and evaluation of a user experience questionnaire* (pp. 63–76). Symposium of the Austrian HCI and Usability Engineering Group.

Lee, J. D., & Moray, N. (1992). Trust, control strategies and allocation of function in human-machine systems. *Ergonomics, 35*, 1243–1270. https://10.1080/00140139208967392

Lee, J. D., & Moray, N. (1994). Trust, self-confidence, and operators' adaptation to automation. *International Journal of Human-Computer Studies, 40*, 153–184. https://doi.org/10.1006/ijhc.1994.1007

Madsen, M., & Gregor, S. (2000). Measuring human-computer trust. *11th Australasian Conference on Information Systems, 53*, 6–8.

Malle, B. F., & Ullman, D. (2021). A multi-dimensional conception and measure of human-robot trust. In C. S. Nam & J. B. Lyons (Eds.), *Trust in human-robot interaction: Research and applications* (pp. 3–25). Academic Press.

Mayer, R. C., & Davis, J. H. (1999). The effect of the performance appraisal system on trust for management: A field quasi-experiment. *Journal of Applied Psychology, 84*, 123. https://doi.org/10.1037/0021-9010.84.1.123

McGlynn, S. A., Kemple, S., Mitzner, T. L., King, C. A., & Rogers, W. A. (2017). Understanding the potential of PARO for healthy older adults. *International Journal of Human-Computer Studies, 100*, 33–47. https://doi.org/10.1016/j.ijhcs.2016.12.004

Merritt, S. M. (2011). Affective processes in human–automation interactions. *Human Factors, 53*, 356–370. https://doi.org/10.1177/0018720811411912

Mitzner, T. L., Tiberio, L., Kemp, C. C., & Rogers, W. A. (2018). Understanding healthcare providers' perceptions of a personal assistant robot. *Gerontechnology, 17*(1), 48–55. https://doi.org/10.4017/gt.2018.17.1.005.00

Moulaei, K., Moulaei, R., & Bahaadinbeigy, K. (2024). The most used questionnaires for evaluating the usability of robots and smart wearables: A scoping review. *Digital Health, 10*, 20552076241237384. https://doi.org/10.1177/20552076241237384

Muir, B. M., & Moray, N. (1996). Experimental studies of trust and human intervention in a process control simulation. *Ergonomics, 39*, 429–460. https://doi.org/10.1080/00140139608964474

Nomura, T., Suzuki, T., Kanda, T., & Kato, K. (2006). Measurement of negative attitudes toward robots. *Interaction Studies, 7*, 437e454.

Olatunji, S. A., Nguyen, V., Cakmak, M., Edsinger, A., Kemp, C. C., Rogers, W. A., & Mahajan, H. P. (2024). Immersive participatory design of assistive robots to support older adults. *Ergonomics, 67*, 6, 717–731. https://doi.org/10.1080/00140139.2024.2312529

Phillips, E., Zhao, X., Ullman, D., & Malle, B. F. (2018). What is human-like? Decomposing robot human-like appearance using the Anthropomorphic roBOT (ABOT) Database. HRI '18, Chicago, IL, USA.

Rogers, W. A., Kadylak, T., & Bayles, M. A. (2022). Maximizing the benefits of participatory design for human-robot interaction research with older adults. *Human Factors, 64*(3), 441–450. https://doi.org/10.1177/00187208211037465

Rogers, W. A., & Mitzner, T. L. (2015). *Survey instruments for robotics research in the Human Factors and Aging Laboratory (HFA-TR-1501)*. Atlanta: Georgia Institute of Technology, School of Psychology, Human Factors and Aging Laboratory.

Schaefer, K. E. (2016). Measuring trust in human robot interactions: Development of the "trust perception scale-HRI." In R. Mittu, D. Sofge, A. Wagner, & W. F. Lawless (Eds.), *Robust intelligence and trust in autonomous systems* (pp. 191–218). Springer.

Singh, I. L., Molloy, R., & Parasuraman, R. (1993). Automation-induced "complacency": Development of the complacency-potential rating scale. *The International Journal of Aviation Psychology, 3*, 111–122. https://doi.org/10.1207/s15327108ijap0302_2

Smarr, C. A., Mitzner, T. L., Beer, J. M., Prakash, A. Chen, T. L., Kemp, C. C., & Rogers, W. A. (2014). Domestic robots for older adults: Attitudes, preferences, and potential. *International Journal of Social Robotics, 6*(2), 229–247.

Steinfeld, A., Jenkins, O. C., & Scassellati, B. (2009). The Oz of Wizard: Simulating the human for interaction research. *2009 4th ACM/IEEE International Conference on Human-Robot Interaction (HRI)*, San Diego, CA, USA (pp. 101–107).

Stroessner, S. J., & Benitez, J. (2019). The social perception of humanoid and non-humanoid robots: Effects of gendered and machinelike features. *International Journal of Social Robotics, 11*(2), 305–315. https://doi.org/10.1007/s12369-018-0502-7

TechSAge (2017). TechSAge Tool: Personas for designing for individuals aging with mobility impairment. Rehabilitation Engineering Research Center on Technologies to Support Aging-in-Place for People with Long-Term Disabilities. https://techsage.gatech.edu/sites/default/files/2021-01/Design%20Personas%20TS%20Tool_0.pdf

Vargas, C., Whelan, J., Brimblecombe, J., & Allender, S. (2022). Co-creation, co-design and co-production for public health: A perspective on definitions and distinctions. *Public Health Research and Practice, 32*(2), e3222211. https://doi.org/10.17061/phrp3222211

Wojton, H. M., Porter, D., Lane, S. T., Bieber, C., and Madhavan, P. (2020). Initial validation of the trust of automated systems test (TOAST). *Journal of Social Psychology, 160*, 735–750. https://doi.org/10.1080/00224545.2020.1749020

Chapter 8

Borenstein, J., & Pearson, Y. (2012). Robot caregivers: Ethical issues across the human lifespan. In P. Lin, K. Abney, & G. Bekey (Eds.), *The ethical and social implications of robots* (pp. 251–265). MIT Press.

Kadylak, T., Bayles, M. A., & Rogers, W. A. (2023). Are friendly robots trusted more? An analysis of robot sociability and trust. *Robotics, 12*, 162. https://doi.org/10.3390/robotics12060162

Kemp, C. C., Edsinger, A., Clever, H. M., & Matulevich, B. (2022). The design of Stretch: A compact, lightweight mobile manipulator for indoor human environments. *International Conference on Robotics and Automation* (ICRA) (pp. 3150–3157). IEEE.

Law, M., Baptiste, S., & Carswell, A. (2019). *COPM manual: Canadian occupational performance measure* (5th ed.). COPM Inc.

Nguyen, V., Cakmak, M., Fair-Field, T., Rogers, W. A. & Kemp, C. C. (under review). Beyond motor impairment: Empowering functional performance with robotics. *Occupational Therapy Journal of Research.*

Olatunji, S. A., Nguyen, V., Cakmak, M., Edsinger, A., Kemp, C. C., Rogers, W. A., & Mahajan, H. P. (2024). Immersive participatory design of assistive robots to support older adults. *Ergonomics, 67*, 717–731. https://doi.org/10.1080/00140139.2024.2312529

Olatunji, S. A., Nguyen, V., Cao, Y., Evans, H., Evans, J., Edsinger, A., Kemp, C. C., & Rogers, W. A. (2023). Advancing the design of trustworthy robots for older adults in home environments: A participatory design approach. *Proceedings of the Human Factors and Ergonomics Society Annual Meeting, 67*(1), 2545–2551. https://doi.org/10.1177/21695067231205566

Ranganeni, V., Nguyen, V., Evans, H., Evans, J., Mehu, J., Olatunji, S., Rogers, W., Edsinger, A., Kemp, C., & Cakmak, M. (2024). Robots for humanity: In-home deployment of Stretch RE2. In *ACM/IEEE International Conference on Human-Robot Interaction* (pp. 1299–1301). https://doi.org/10.1145/3610978.3641114

Chapter 9

Czaja, S. J., & Sharit, J. (2012). *Designing training and instructional programs for older adults*. CRC Press.

Davis, F. (1989). Perceived usefulness, perceived ease of use, and user acceptance of information technology. *MIS Quarterly, 13*, 319–340. https://doi.org/10.2307/249008

Felding, S. A., Koh, W. Q., Teupen, S., Budak, K. B., Uribel, F. L., & Roes, M. (2023). A scoping review using the Almere Model to understand factors facilitating and hindering the acceptance of social robots in nursing homes. *International Journal of Social Robotics, 15,* 1115–1153. https://doi.org/10.1007/s12369-023-01012-1

Fisk, A. D. (1999). Human factors and the older adult. *Ergonomics in Design, 7(1)*, 8–13. https://doi.org/10.1177/106480469900700103

Glasgow, R. E., & Estabrooks, P. E. (2018). Pragmatic applications of RE-AIM for health care initiatives in community and clinical settings. *Preventing Chronic Disease, 15,* E02. https://doi.org/10.5888/pcd15.170271

Heerink, M., Kröse, B., Evers, V., & Wielinga, B. (2010). Assessing acceptance of assistive social agent technology by older adults: The Almere model. *International Journal of Social Robotics,* 2(4), 361–375. https://doi.org/10.1007/s12369-010-0068-5

Mois, G., & Rogers, W. A. (2024). Developing a framework for digital activities of daily living. *The Gerontologist, 64*(10), gnae110. https://doi.org/10.1093/geront/gnae110

Ory, M. G., Altpeter, M., Belza, B., Helduser, J., Zhang, C., & Smith, M. L. (2015). Perceived utility of the RE-AIM framework for health promotion/disease prevention initiatives for older adults: A case study from the U.S. evidence-based disease prevention initiative. *Frontiers in Public Health,* 2(143). https://doi.org/10.3389/fpubh.2014.00143

Rogers, E. M. (2003). *Diffusion of innovations* (5th ed.). Simon & Schuster.

Venkatesh, V., Thong, J. Y., L., & Xu, X. (2012). Consumer acceptance and use of information technology: Extending the unified theory of acceptance and use of technology. *MIS Quarterly, 36*, 157–178.

Chapter 10

Mintrom, M., Sumartojo, S., Kulić, D., Tian, L., Carreno-Medrano, P., & Allen, A. (2021). Robots in public spaces: Implications for policy design. *Policy Design and Practice, 5*(2), 123–139. https://doi.org/10.1080/25741292.2021.1905342

Rogers, W. A., & Mitzner, T. L. (2017). Envisioning the future for older adults: Autonomy, health, well-being, and social connectedness with technology support. *Futures, 87*, 133–139. https://doi.org/10.1016/j.futures.2016.07.002

Index

Note: **Bold** page numbers refer to tables and *italic* page numbers refer to figures.